Handbook on Adverse Drug Reactions in TB Treatment

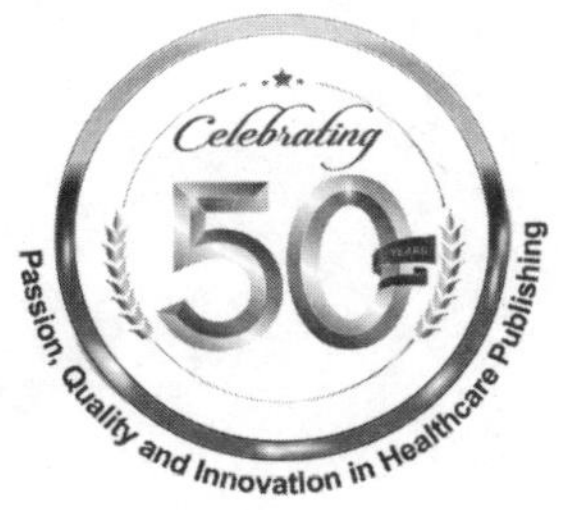

Handbook on Adverse Drug Reactions in TB Treatment

Author

Rajendra Prasad MD DTCD FAMS FCCP (USA) FRCP (Glasgow) FNCCP FICS FCAI FIAB FIMSA FCCS DSc (Honoris Causa)

Director, Medical Education
Professor and Head
Department of Pulmonary Medicine
Era's Lucknow Medical College and Hospital
Era University
Lucknow, Uttar Pradesh, India

Formerly

Director, Vallabhbhai Patel Chest Institute
University of Delhi
New Delhi, India

Professor and Head, Department of Pulmonary Medicine
King George's Medical University
Lucknow, Uttar Pradesh, India

Director, UP Rural Institute of Medical Sciences and Research
Saifai, Etawah, Uttar Pradesh, India

Co-author

Nikhil Gupta MD (Medicine)

Assistant Professor
Department of General Medicine
Dr Ram Manohar Lohia Institute of Medical Sciences
Lucknow, Uttar Pradesh, India

Foreword

D Behera

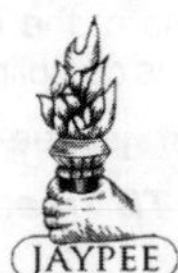

JAYPEE BROTHERS MEDICAL PUBLISHERS

The Health Sciences Publisher

New Delhi | London | Panama

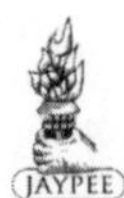

Jaypee Brothers Medical Publishers (P) Ltd

Headquarters

Jaypee Brothers Medical Publishers (P) Ltd
4838/24, Ansari Road, Daryaganj
New Delhi 110 002, India
Phone: +91-11-43574357
Fax: +91-11-43574314
Email: jaypee@jaypeebrothers.com

Overseas Offices

J.P. Medical Ltd
83 Victoria Street, London
SW1H 0HW (UK)
Phone: +44 20 3170 8910
Fax: +44 (0)20 3008 6180
Email: info@jpmedpub.com

Jaypee-Highlights Medical Publishers Inc
City of Knowledge, Bld. 235, 2nd Floor, Clayton
Panama City, Panama
Phone: +1 507-301-0496
Fax: +1 507-301-0499
Email: cservice@jphmedical.com

Jaypee Brothers Medical Publishers (P) Ltd
17/1-B Babar Road, Block-B, Shyamoli
Mohammadpur, Dhaka-1207
Bangladesh
Mobile: +08801912003485
Email: jaypeedhaka@gmail.com

Jaypee Brothers Medical Publishers (P) Ltd
Bhotahity, Kathmandu
Nepal
Phone: +977-9741283608
Email: kathmandu@jaypeebrothers.com

Website: www.jaypeebrothers.com
Website: www.jaypeedigital.com

Inquiries for bulk sales may be solicited at: jaypee@jaypeebrothers.com

Handbook on Adverse Drug Reactions in TB Treatment

First Edition: ***2019***

ISBN: 978-93-5270-106-3

Printed at Rajkamal Electric Press, Kundli, Haryana.

Dedicated to

My teachers for their guidance, wisdom and inspiration

and

My parents, wife and children for their love and patience

"संस्थान में हिंदी पत्रों का स्वागत है"
श्वास रोग चिकित्सा विभाग
स्नातकोत्तर चिकित्सा शिक्षा एवं अनुसंधान संस्थान, चण्डीगढ़ – १६० ०१२ (भारत)
DEPARTMENT OF PULMONARY MEDICINE
(WHO Collaborating Centre for Research & Capacity Building in Chronic Respiratory Diseases)
POSTGRADUATE INSTITUTE OF MEDICAL EDUCATION & RESEARCH, CHANDIGARH-160012 (INDIA)
डॉ. दिगम्बर बेहेरा
प्राचार्य एव विभागाध्यक्ष
Dr. Digambar Behera
M.D.(Med.), FCCP, FAMS, FNCCP, FICP, FICA, FAPSR,
FICS, MNAMS (Med.). Dip. NBE (Resp. Med.)
Professor (Sr. Scale) & Head
Prof. Incharge (Engineering)

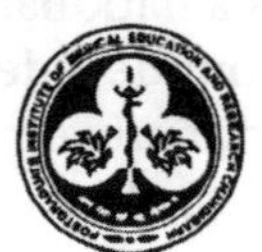

Foreword

Tuberculosis is a multisystem disease with varied clinical presentations. It has reached epidemic proportions and has tormented mankind for centuries with impact on human beings unparalleled in the history of communicable diseases. One-third of the world's population is infected with *Mycobacterium tuberculosis* and there is 10% lifetime risk of developing tuberculosis and the risk further increases to 10% annual risk in immunocompromised patients. Globally, it was responsible for causing 1.8 million deaths in the year 2015 out of which 0.51 million deaths occurred in India alone. Additionally, the increasing burden of multidrug-resistant (MDR-TB) and extensively drug-resistant tuberculosis (XDR-TB) is posing challenge to tuberculosis control.

Globally, attempts are being made to prevent, reduce and better management of adverse drug reactions in treatment of tuberculosis through increased awareness of healthcare workers, doctors, patients and their family. Adequate prevention, early recognition and management of adverse drug reactions are considered to be important in tuberculosis treatment as poor management can result in increased morbidity, mortality and non-compliance leading to drug resistance.

Against this backdrop, the publication of *Handbook on Adverse Drug Reactions in TB Treatment* by Professor Rajendra Prasad is a timely and useful addition to the existing literature. The book summarizes the current status or knowledge on every aspect of adverse drug reactions in tuberculosis treatment. There are 21 chapters in the handbook. Chapters practically cover all the aspects of adverse drug reactions in tuberculosis treatment ranging from pharmacology, interaction between anti-TB drugs with food and other drugs including antiretroviral drugs, monitoring and management of adverse drug reactions of antituberculosis drugs used in new and drug resistant cases of tuberculosis. The chapters in the book have been arranged in a systematic sequence for easy understanding and are based on practical approach with illustrative cases, blended with the most up-to-date knowledge in the field. The chapters have been written on the basis of vast and rich clinical experience gained by the author from day-to-day patient management over the last four decades.

Professor Rajendra Prasad is a nationally acclaimed chest physician and tuberculosis expert, possessing four decades of illustrious teaching, research and administrative experience with proven excellence in quality patient care. Apart from being a clinician par excellence, he is also a very popular medical teacher in pulmonary medicine. He is currently Director, Medical Education, Professor and Head, Era's Lucknow Medical College and Hospital, Lucknow, Uttar Pradesh, India. He has earlier served as Director of Vallabhbhai Patel Chest Institute, Delhi, India, Professor and Head, Department of Pulmonary Medicine, King George's Medical University, Lucknow, and Director, UP Rural Institute of Medical Sciences and Research, Saifai, Etawah, Uttar Pradesh. He has devoted all his energy in promoting medical education, patient care and research. His contribution in the field of tuberculosis and multidrug-resistant tuberculosis (MDR-TB) are widely acclaimed. He took keen interest in Revised National Tuberculosis Control Program (RNTCP) from its inception. His dynamic leadership in academic, patient care and administrative areas has earned him a large number of awards from various international and national scientific societies including prestigious Dr BC Roy National Award.

This comprehensive well-referenced handbook contains a plethora of knowledge and would be a valuable source for undergraduate and postgraduate medical students, clinicians, healthcare workers caring for patients of tuberculosis. I am quite hopeful that his handbook will help in better understanding towards alleviating the suffering of millions from tuberculosis. This handbook deserves a place in the library of every medical college and healthcare providing institutions.

D Behera
Chairman
National Task Force for Involvement of Medical Colleges under RNTCP
Chairman
National Operational Research Committee, RNTCP
Ex-Director
National Institute of TB and Respiratory Diseases
(Previously LRS Institute), New Delhi, India

Preface

As a senior author of this book, I look upon tuberculosis as a 100% curable disease throughout the 40 years of my clinical practice in pulmonary medicine, provided adequate regimen is prescribed by doctor and taken by patients. Practically, there should be no relapse, drug resistance and death. However, tuberculosis still continues to be the world's most important infectious cause of morbidity and mortality. Globally, there were an estimated 10.4 million new cases of tuberculosis causing death to 1.8 million people in 2015. In India, there were an estimated 2.8 million (27% of the total cases) new cases causing death to 0.48 million people due to tuberculosis in 2015. It is a cause for concern as India stands first in terms of absolute number of cases. It is a real paradox because pathogenesis, transmission, prevention, diagnosis, and treatment are well known for tuberculosis. Drug-resistant tuberculosis has been reported since the early days of introduction of anti-TB chemotherapy but multidrug-resistant tuberculosis (MDR-TB), extensively drug-resistant tuberculosis (XDR-TB), and most recently total drug-resistant tuberculosis (TDR-TB) has been an area of growing concern and is posing threat to global efforts of tuberculosis control.

Globally, attempts are being made to prevent, reduce and better management of adverse drug reaction in treatment of tuberculosis through increased awareness of healthcare workers, doctors, patients and their family. Adequate prevention, early recognition and management of adverse drug reaction is considered to be important in tuberculosis treatment as poor management can result in increased morbidity, mortality and non compliance leading to drug resistance.

This book is written with the aim of defining a practical approach to every aspect of adverse drug reaction in tuberculosis treatment. In total, there are 21 chapters in the book. Chapters practically cover all the aspects of adverse drug reaction in TB treatment ranging from pharmacology, interaction between anti-TB drugs with food and other drugs including antiretroviral drugs, monitoring and management of adverse drug reaction of antituberculosis used in new and drug-resistant cases of tuberculosis. Special chapters on case-based approach to treatment of tuberculosis and MDR-TB and XDR-TB in special situation like pregnancy, renal insufficiency and liver diseases and epidemiology of adverse drug reactions in new and drug-resistant patients of tuberculosis have also been included. Chapters have been written in the background of current literature and practical experience gained from day-to-day dealing with different patients suffering from tuberculosis. Advances up to 2016 have been included making all the chapters well referenced with the latest references.

This book will be useful to both undergraduate and postgraduate medical students, practitioners and program managers and healthcare workers. In total, this book will serve as a very useful practical guide regarding all aspects of adverse drug reactions in tuberculosis treatment.

Rajendra Prasad

Acknowledgments

As a senior author of this book, I wish to acknowledge my indebtedness to a number of people who significantly contributed to the publication of this book. The individual to whom I would like to acknowledge first is Prof BK Khanna who as a Head of Department of Tuberculosis at the King George's Medical College, Lucknow, Uttar Pradesh, India, while I was postgraduate student in that department, markedly stimulated my interest in tuberculosis. Prof BK Khanna's own tremendous knowledge and wisdom in the field of tuberculosis set an example of thoughtfulness and meticulousness which I have always tried to emulate. I am also indebted to Prof PK Mukherjee, Late Dr MS Agnihotri, Late Dr Jafar Jameel and Late Dr J Nath, for their great inspiration as teachers during my postgraduate days. I am greatly indebted to many postgraduate students who have been trained with me in the department at King George's Medical College, Lucknow; Vallabhbhai Patel Chest Institute, Delhi, India, and Era's Lucknow Medical College and Hospital, Lucknow, especially Dr Sanjay Verma, Dr Kiran Vishnu Narayan, Dr Suneesh C Anand, Dr Giridhar BH, Dr Abhijeet, Dr Abhishek Agrawal, Dr Shailendra Singh, Dr Mandeep Singh, Dr Pawan Gupta, Dr Visweswaran Balasubramanian, Dr Faizan Ahmad, Dr Amitabh Banka, Dr Sakshi Batra, Dr Ronal Naorem, and Dr Asna Khan. The efforts of these postgraduate students in part is responsible for generating much of the data that can be incorporated in making the chapters in book more evidence based.

I also wish to express my appreciation to Dr Nikhil Gupta, co-author of this book, for helping me in preparing and correcting the manuscript. I also wish to express my thanks to Mr PP Sharma, Mr Ashish Yadav, Mr Gyan Prakash, Mr Mithun, and Miss Seema Shukla for their invaluable help in the preparation and typing of manuscript. I am also thankful to all my patients, who gave me experience in the field of tuberculosis.

I am very grateful to the whole team of M/s Jaypee Brothers Medical Publishers (P) Ltd, who helped and guided me, Shri Jitendar P Vij (Group Chairman), Mr Ankit Vij (Managing Director), Ms Ritu Sharma (Director–Content Strategy), Ms Pooja Bhandari (Production Head), Ms Sunita Katla (PA to Group Chairman and Publishing Manager) and team members for all their support to work in this project and make it a success. Without their cooperation, I could not have completed this project.

Contents

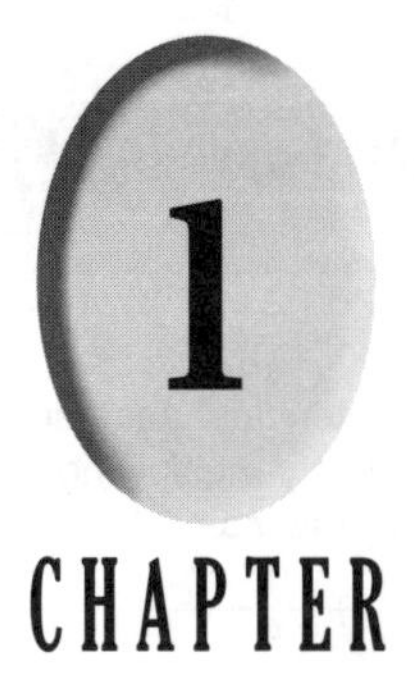

CHAPTER

Antitubercular Drug Doses and Regimens for Adults and Children

Antitubercular drugs with their doses used in new and previously treated patients of tuberculosis are tabulated in Tables 1.1, 1.2 and 1.3.

TABLE 1.1: Dose of antitubercular drugs used in new patients of tuberculosis.

Drugs	Daily		Intermittent	
	Adult	Children*	3-weekly	2-weekly
H	5 (4–6)	10 (10–15)	10 (8–12)	15 (13–17)
R	10 (8–12)	15 (10–20)	10 (8–12)	10 (8–12)
Z	25 (20–30)	35 (30–40)	35 (30–40)	50 (40–60)
E	15 (15–20)	20 (15–25)	30 (25–35)	45 (40–50)
S	15 (12–18)	15 (12–18)	15 (12–18)	15 (12–18)

*Doses modified in 2008.
(H: isoniazid; R: rifampicin; Z: pyrazinamide; E: ethambutol, S: streptomycin).

TABLE 1.2: Doses of antitubercular drugs used in previously treated tuberculosis patients

Drugs	Average daily dosage	Daily dosage (mg)		Type of anti-mycobacterial activity
		Minimum	Maximum	
Group 1 First line oral agents				
Pyrazinamide (Z)	25 mg/kg	1,200	1,500	Bactericidal
Ethambutol (E)	15 mg/kg	800	1,200	Bacteriostatic
Rifabutin (Rfb)	5–10 mg/kg	150	600	Bactericidal

(Contd.)

(Contd.)

Drugs	Average daily dosage	Daily dosage (mg)		Type of anti-mycobacterial activity
		Minimum	Maximum	
Group 2 **Injectable agents** Kanamycin (Km) Amikacin (Am) Streptomycin (S) Capreomycin (Cm)	 15 mg/kg 15 mg/kg 15 mg/kg 15 mg/kg	 750 750 750 750	 1,000 1,000 1,000 1,000	 Bactericidal against actively multiplying organisms
Group 3 **Oral bacteriostatic second line drugs** Ethionamide (Eto) Prothionamide (Pto) Para-aminosalicylic acid (PAS) Cycloserine (Cs) Terizidone (Trd)	 15–20 mg/kg 15–20 mg/kg 200–300 mg/kg 10–20 mg/kg 10–20 mg/kg	 500–750 500–750 10 g 500–750 500–750	 1,000 1,000 12 g 1,000 1,000	 Bacteriostatic
Group 4 **Fluoroquinolone** Moxifloxacin (Mfx) Ofloxacin (Ofx) Levofloxacin (Lfx)	 7.5–10 mg/kg 15–20 mg/kg 7.5–10 mg/kg	 400 800 500	 400 1,000 1,000	 Weakly bactericidal
Group 5 **Agents with unclear role in treatment of drug resistant TB** Clofazimine (Cfz) Linezolid (Lzd) Amoxicillin/clavulanate (Amx/Clv) Thioacetazone (Thz) Imipenem/cilastatin (Ipm/Cln) High dose isoniazid (high-dose H) Clarithromycin (Clr)	 4–5 mg/kg - 2 g/day 150 mg/day 500–1,000 mg/kg/IV every 6 hourly 16–20 mg/kg 10–15 mg/kg	 100 600 500/125 twice a day - 500 600 500 twice a day	 300 600 1,000/250 twice a day - 1,000 900 500 twice a day	 Bacteriostatic Weakly bactericidal Bactericidal (pH dependent)

TABLE 1.3: Doses of antitubercular drugs used in drug resistant tuberculosis patients (WHO-2016).

Groups	Drugs	Average daily dose	Daily dosage (mg)	
			Minimum	Maximum
A. Fluoroquinolones	Levofloxacin Moxifloxacin Gatifloxacin	7.5–10 mg/kg 7.5–10 mg/kg 7.5–10 mg/kg	750 400 400	1000 400 400

(Contd.)

(Contd.)

Groups		Drugs	Average daily dose	Daily dosage (mg)	
				Minimum	Maximum
B. Second line injectable agents		Amikacin Kanamycin Capreomycin Streptomycin	15 mg/kg 15 mg/kg 15 mg/kg 15 mg/kg	500 500 500 500	1,000 1,000 1,000 1,000
C. Other core second line agent		Ethionamide/ prothionamide Cycloserine/ terizidone Linezolid Clofazimine	15–20 mg/kg 10–20 mg/kg - 4–5 mg/kg	500 500 600 100	1,000 1,000 600 300
D. Add on agents	D1	Pyrazinamide Ethambutol High dose isoniazid	25 mg/kg 15 mg/kg 16–20 mg/kg	750 600 600	2,000 1,200 1,500
	D2	Bedaquiline	400 mg OD x 2 weeks and then 200 mg 3 times per week		
		Delamanid	100 mg twice daily		
	D3	PAS	200–300 mg/ kg	10 g	12 g
		Imipenem-cilastatin	1,000 mg/1,000 mg twice daily		
		Meropenem	1,000 mg thrice daily		
		Amoxicillin-clavulanate	80 mg/kg/day	500/125 mg BD	1000/250 mg BD
		Thioacetazone	150 mg once daily		

World Health Organization (WHO) recommended treatment regimens for each diagnostic category for adults and children are tabulated in Tables 1.4 and 1.5. Various standard chemotherapy regimens for newly diagnosed patents of tuberculosis by international union against tuberculosis and lung disease are tabulated in Table 1.6. New WHO guideline (2009) for treatment of tuberculosis is tabulated in Table 1.7.

TABLE 1.4: Revised National Tuberculosis Control Program (RNTCP) treatment regimen (Technical and operational guideline for TB control in India 2016).

TB patients	TB treatment regimens	
	Initial phase[a]	Continuation phase
New patients	2 HRZE[b]	4 HRE
Previously treated patients	2 HRZES/1 HRZE	5 HRE
Rifampicin resistant +isoniazid sensitive or unknown	(6–9) Km Z E Eto Cs Lfx H	18 Eto Cs Lfx E H

(Contd.)

(Contd.)

TB patients	TB treatment regimens	
	Initial phase[a]	Continuation phase
Confirmed MDR-TB patients	(6–9) Km Z E Eto Cs Lfx (modify treatment based on the level of INH resistance)[c]	18 Eto Cs Lfx E
Confirmed XDR-TB patients	(6–12) Cm PAS Mfx High dose-H Cfz Lzd Amx/Clv	18 PAS Mfx High dose-H Cfz Lzd Amx/Clv

(H: isoniazid; Z: pyrazinamide; E: ethambutol; Rfb: rifabutin; Km: kanamycin; Am: amikacin; S: streptomycin; Cm: capreomycin; Mfx: moxifloxacin; Lfx: levofloxacin; Eto: ethionamide; Pto: prothionamide; PAS: para-aminosalicylic acid; Cs: cycloserine; Trd: terizidone; Cfz: clofazimine; Lzd: linezolid; Amx/Clv: amoxicillin/clavulanate; Thz: thiacetazone; Ipm/Cln: imipenem/cilastatin; high-dose H: high dose isoniazid; Clr: clarithromycin)

[a] Direct observation of drug intake is required during the initial phase of treatment in smear-positive cases and always in treatment that includes rifampicin.

[b] In tubercular meningitis (TBM), spinal TB with neurological complications and other hematogenous tuberculosis continuation phase may be extended for 12–24 months based on clinical decision of the treating physician.

[c] For isoniazid resistance, decision of use of isoniazid in the regimen depends on the following:

- If high level resistance detected by liquid culture — omit INH
- If low level resistance detected by liquid culture — add high dose of INH
- If LPA reports INH resistance by Kat G mutation — omit INH
- If LPA reports INH resistance by INH A mutation — use high dose INH. Ethionamide in the treatment regimen may be replaced with PAS

TABLE 1.5: WHO treatment categories and regimen for children 2014.

TB diagnostic category	Anti-TB drug regimen	
	Intensive phase	Continuation phase
Low HIV prevalence (and HIV-negative children) and low isoniazid resistance settings		
Smear-negative pulmonary TB Intrathoracic lymph node TB Tuberculous peripheral lymphadenitis	2 HRZ	4 HR
Extensive pulmonary disease Smear-positive pulmonary TB Severe forms of extrapulmonary TB (other than tuberculous meningitis/osteoarticular TB)	2 HRZE	4 HR
High HIV prevalence or high isoniazid resistance or both		
Smear-positive PTB Smear-negative PTB with or without extensive parenchymal disease All forms of EPTB except tuberculous meningitis and osteoarticular TB	2 HRZE	4 HR
All regions		
Tuberculous meningitis and osteoarticular TB	2 HRZE	10 HR
MDR-TB	Individualized regimen	

(E: ethambutol; H: isoniazid; R: rifampicin; Z: pyrazinamide)

TABLE 1.6: Various standard chemotherapy for newly diagnosed patient.

Recommended standard 6-month regimen	
• 2 EHRZ/4 HR • 2 HRZ/4 HR	• 2 SHRZ/4 HR
Variants of standard 6-month regimen (supervised chemotherapy)	
• 2 HRZ/4 H_3R_3 • 2 $E_3H_3Z_3$/4 H_3R_3 • 2 $E_3H_3R_3Z_3$/4 H_3R_3	• 2 HRZ/4 H_2R_2 • 2 $S_3H_3R_3Z_3$/4 H_3R_3
Alternative less potent regimens of longer duration	
1. With a potent initial 4-drug phase • 2 SHRZ/6 HT or 6 HE	• 2 SHRZ/6 $S_2H_2Z_2$
2. With a less potent or no initial phase • 2 SHR/7 HR • 9 HR • 2 SHE/10 • 12 HT or 12 HE	• 2 HER/7 HR • 2 SHT/10 HT • 2 SHP/10 HP • 12 S_2H_2

(S: streptomycin; H: isoniazid; R: rifampicin; Z: pyrazinamide; E: ethambutol; T: thiocetazone; P: para-aminosalicylic acid)

TABLE 1.7: Treatment of TB (WHO 2009 guidelines).

New patient regimen	Retreatment regimen with first line drugs	MDR regimen
1. Should receive a regimen containing 6 months of rifampicin: 2 HRZE/4 HR 2. Should receive a regimen containing 6 months of rifampicin along with ethambutol: 2 HRZE/4 HRE where high levels of isoniazid resistance in new TB patients is suspected (presence of resistance to low concentrations of isoniazid (>1% of bacilli resistant to 0.2 µg/mL but susceptible to 1 µg/mL of isoniazid) 3. Should receive daily TB treatment at least during the intensive phase or for the continuation phase, the optimal dosing frequency is also daily for these TB patients with known positive HIV status and also living in HIV-prevalent settings (defined as countries, subnational administrative units, or selected facilities where the HIV prevalence among adult pregnant women is ≥1% or among TB patients is ≥5%)	1. TB patients returning after *defaulting* or *relapsing* from their first treatment course may receive the retreatment regimen containing first-line drugs 2 HRZES/1 HRZE/5 HRE if country-specific data show low or medium levels of MDR in these patients or if such data are not available 2. Should receive daily TB treatment rather than intermittent treatment	1. Use at least 4 drugs certain to be effective 2. Do not use drugs for which there is the possibility of cross- resistance 3. Eliminate drugs that are not safe 4. Include drugs from Groups 1–5 in a hierarchical order based on potency. For further details see chapter on MDR-TB

FURTHER READINGS

1. Companion Handbook to the WHO guidelines for the programmatic management of drug resistant tuberculosis. WHO/HTM/TB/2014.11.
2. Guidelines for programmatic management of drug resistant tuberculosis. WHO, 2011. WHO/HTM/TB/2011.6
3. Guidelines for the programmatic management of drug-resistant tuberculosis: emergency update 2008. Geneva, World Health Organization, 2008 (WHO/HTM/TB/ 2008.402).
4. International Union Against Tuberculosis and Lung Disease. Management of tuberculosis: a guide for low income countries. Fifth edition. Paris: IUATLD;2000.
5. International Union Against Tuberculosis and Lung Diseases. Guidelines for Clinical and Operational Management of Drug-Resistant Tuberculosis. Paris: IUTLD; 2013.
6. Jindani A, Nunn AJ, Enarson DA. Two 8-month regimens of chemotherapy for treatment of newly diagnosed pulmonary tuberculosis: international multicentre randomised trial. Lancet. 2004;364:1244-51.
7. Management of patients with multidrug resistant/extensively drug-resistant tuberculosis in Europe: a TBNET consensus statement. E R J. 2014; 44:23-63.
8. Nahid P, et al. ATS/CDC/IDSA Clinical Practice Guidelines: Treatment of Drug-Susceptible Tuberculosis. Clin Infec Dis. 2016:1-50.
9. Technical and Operational Guidelines for TB Control in India 2016.
10. Treatment of tuberculosis: guidelines for national programmes, 3rd edition Geneva, World Health Organization, 2003 (WHO/CDS/TB/2003.313).
11. WHO treatment guidelines for Drug-Resistent Tuberculosis – 2016 Update. WHO/HTM/TB/2016.04.
12. World Health Organization. Guidance for National Tuberculosis and HIV Programmes on the management of tuberculosis in HIV-infected children: recommendations for a public health approach. Geneva: World Health Organization; 2010.
13. World Health Organization. Guidance for national tuberculosis programmes on the management of tuberculosis in children 2006 and 2014.
14. World Health Organization. Report of the meeting on TB medicines for children-July 2008. World Health Organization, Geneva; 2008.
15. World Health Organization. Treatment of TB Guidelines - 4th edition. WHO/HTM/TB/2009.420.

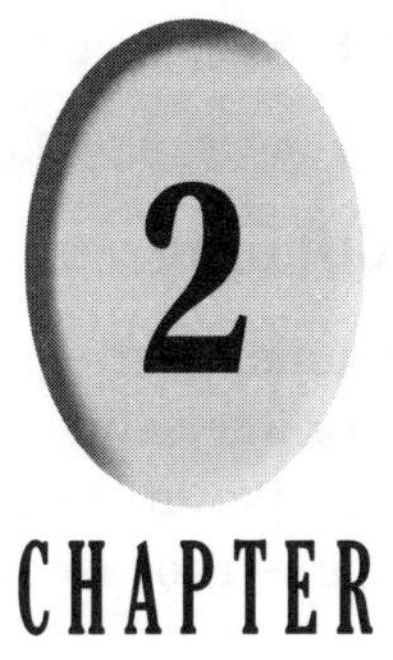

CHAPTER 2 Duration of Treatment in Tuberculosis

In general, optimal duration of treatment for various short course regimes is 6–9 months and for standard conventional long-term regimes (without rifampicin) is 1–2 years (Table 2.1).

TABLE 2.1: Duration of treatment in different regimens.

If Z is used during intensive phase—6 months
2 RHEZ/4 RH 2 RHZ/4RH 2 SHRZ/4 RH
If continuation phase is without R—8 months
2 RHEZ/6 EH/TH 2 RHZ/6 EH/TH 2 SHRZ/6 EH/TH
If Z is not used in intensive phase—9 months
2 RHE/7 RH 9 RHE
If R and Z is not used — 1–2 years
2 STH/10 TH 2 SHE/10 HE 12 TH
Such duration is enough for pulmonary tuberculosis as well as extrapulmonary tuberculosis

(H: isoniazid; R: rifampicin; Z: pyrazinamide; E: ethambutol; S: streptomycin; T: thioacetazone.)

Note: In meningeal TB, ethambutol should be replaced by streptomycin. In tubercular meningitis (TBM), spinal TB with neurological complications and other hematogenous tuberculosis continuation phase is prolonged for 3–6 months.

SPUTUM POSITIVE PULMONARY TUBERCULOSIS

Treatment of newly diagnosed smear positive patients containing rifampicin throughout and pyrazinamide in the intensive phase (initial 2–3 months) daily or intermittent should be for 6 months. Treatment should be for 8 months if rifampicin is not used in continuation phase (2 RHEZ/6 HT or HE).

If pyrazinamide is not used in initial intensive phase (RHE/RH), then the treatment duration is for 9 months.

SPUTUM SMEAR NEGATIVE PULMONARY TUBERCULOSIS

Various studies have shown that duration of regimens containing streptomycin, rifampicin, isoniazid and pyrazinamide given daily or intermittently in smear negative patients is at least for 4 months, however, World Health Organization (WHO) recommended at least 6 months regimen for smear negative pulmonary tuberculosis.

STANDARD CONVENTIONAL LONG-TERM NON-RIFAMPICIN CONTAINING REGIMEN

Before rifampicin and pyrazinamide become available, patients were treated for prolonged period. Standard conventional long-term regimen containing streptomycin (S) for initial 8 weeks with isoniazid (H) and thioacetazone (T) (STH) practically achieve bacteriological quinescence within 6 months but about of quarter of patients relapsed in next five years. While there is evidence that more than 18 months of good standard conventional treatment produces no additional benefits in terms of treatment success or prevention of relapse. The optimum duration of streptomycin in conventional long-term regimens is 8 weeks.

FURTHER READINGS

1. American Review results at five year of a controlled comparison of a six months and a standard 18 months regimens of Chemotherapy for pulmonary tuberculosis. American review of Respiratory Diseases. 1977;116:3-8.
2. Controlled clinical trial of 2 months, 3 months and 12 months regimens of chemotherapy for sputum smear negative for pulmonary tuberculosis the result of up to 30 months. Hongkong Chest Service/Tuberculosis Research Center Madras/British Medical Research Council. American Review of Respiratory Diseases. 1981;124:138-142.
3. Controlled clinical trial of four 6 month regimen of chemotherapy for pulmonary tuberculosis IInd report. IInd East African/British Medical Research Council study American review of respiratory disease. 1976;114:471-75.
4. Controlled clinical trials of four short course (6 months) regimen of chemotherapy for treatment of pulmonary tuberculosis. IIIrd report. East African – British Medical Research Council Lancet. 1974;2:237-240.
5. Five year follow up a clinical trial of a three six months regimens of chemotherapy given intermittently in the continuation phase in the treatment of Pulmonary Tuberculosis. Singapore Tuberculosis Service/ British Medical Research Council. American Review of Respiratory Diseases. 1988;137:1147-50.
6. Isoniazid with thiacetazone in the treatment of pulmonary tuberculosis in East African 5th investigation. A cooperative study in East African Hospital, Clinic and laboratories with the collaboration of East African and British Medical Research Council Tubercle. 1970;51:123-151.
7. Nahid P, et al. ATS/CDC/IDSA Clinical Practice Guidelines: Treatment of Drug-Susceptible Tuberculosis. Clin Infec Dis. 2016:1-50.
8. World Health Organization. Treatment of TB Guidelines, 4th edition. WHO/HTM/TB/2009.420.

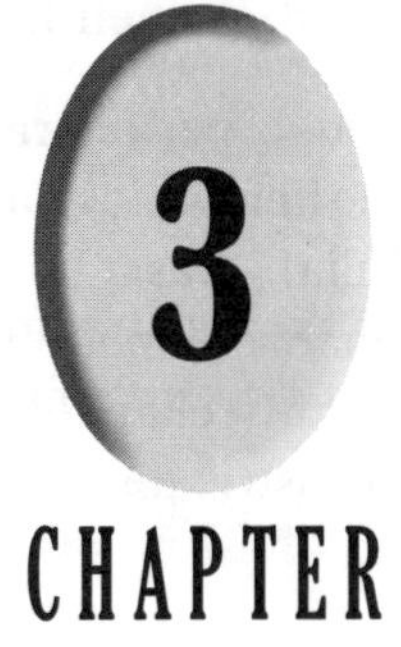

CHAPTER

Pharmacology of Antitubercular Drugs Used in Newly Diagnosed Patients of Tuberculosis

ISONIAZID

It is the hydrazide of isonicotinic acid. It is primarily bactericidal.

Mechanism of Action

It is a prodrug converted into the active drug by mycobacterial catalase-peroxidase. It inhibits the synthesis of mycolic acids which are a part of the mycobacterial cell wall. Resistance to it develops by mutation in at least five of different genes (Kat G, Inh A, Ahp C, Kas A, Ndb), more likely to Inh A.

Distribution

It diffuses readily into all body fluids and cells, e.g. pleural fluid, ascitic, cerebrospinal fluid (CSF) (especially with inflamed meninges), into the caseous material, etc.

Metabolism

It is extensively metabolized in liver, most important pathway being acetylation including fast and slow acetylators.

Excretion

Majority of the dose of isoniazid is excreted in the urine within 24 hours. Excretory products result from enzymatic acetylation and enzymatic hydrolysis.

Preparation and Dose

Isoniazid is supplied in 50 mg, 100 mg and 300 mg tablets or as an elixir containing 50 mg/5 mL. Combined preparations with rifampicin, ethambutol, and pyrazinamide are available. The dose for daily therapy is 5 (4–6) mg/kg, i.e. 300 mg. In twice weekly regimen dosage is 15 (13–17) mg/kg/day and in thrice weekly regimen dosage is 10 (8–12) mg/kg/day.

Side Effects

Common side effects include fever, rash, jaundice (hepatitis), peripheral neuritis and hypersensitivity reaction. Rare side effects include hematological (anemia, thrombocytopenia, agranulocytosis, eosinophilia), vasculitis, neurological disturbances (dizziness, ataxia, toxic encephalopathy), psychiatric disturbances (euphoria, psychosis) and some miscellaneous side effects like dryness of mouth, urinary retention and epigastric distress, gynecomastia.

Renal Disease

Clearance of isoniazid is dependent only to a small degree on the status of renal function but patients who are slow acetylators of the drug may accumulate toxic concentrations if their renal function is impaired.

Pregnancy

Isoniazid is safer in pregnancy.

Contraindications

Isoniazid should not be given in known hypersensitivity and active liver disease.

Overdosage

Overdosage of isoniazid produce nausea, vomiting, dizziness, blurring of vision and slurring of speech. Massive dosage results in unconsciousness followed by respiratory depression and stupor. Severe intractable seizure may occur. Treatment consists of induced emesis, gastric lavage, activated charcoal, antiepileptic and IV sodium bicarbonate. Hemodialysis may be of value. Administration of large doses of pyridoxine is necessary to prevent seizures.

RIFAMPICIN

It is a semi-synthetic-derivative of rifamycin B. It is a bactericidal drug. It is produced by *Streptomyces mediterranei*.

Mechanism of Action

It inhibits DNA dependant RNA synthesis, i.e. it inhibits DNA dependant RNA polymerase of mycobacteria. Rifampicin should be given preferably 30 minutes before the meals since absorption is reduced when the drug is taken with food.

Distribution

Rifampicin is distributed throughout the body and is present in effective concentrations in many organs and body fluids including the CSF. The drug imparts an orange-red color to the urine, feces, saliva, sputum, tears and sweat.

Excretion

The drug is deacetylated in the liver. About 30% of the drug is excreted in urine and about 65% in feces.

Preparation and Dose

Rifampicin is available as capsule or tablets of 150 mg, 300 mg, 450 mg, and 600 mg and as syrup containing 100 mg/5 mL. Combined preparations with isoniazid, and with isoniazid plus pyrazinamide are also available.
The dose for daily therapy being 10 (8–12) mg/kg/day (maximum 600 mg) and it is same in twice or thrice weekly regimen.

Side Effects

Common side effects include gastrointestinal upset (nausea, vomiting, abdominal pain), fever, rash, influenza-like syndrome. Moderate rises in serum concentrations of bilirubin and transaminases are common at the outset of treatment but it is transient and without clinical significance. Dose related hepatitis can also occur but it is less common. Rare side effects include neurological disturbances, hepatitis, hypersensitivity reactions, thrombocytopenia temporary oliguria, exfoliative dermatitis (especially in HIV patients), hemolytic anemia.

Renal Disease

Adjustment of dosage is not necessary in patients with impaired renal function.

Pregnancy

Rifampicin is safer in pregnancy.

Contraindications

Rifampicin is contraindicated in case of hypersensitivity and hepatic dysfunction.

Overdosage

Overdosage of rifampicin can be reverted by gastric lavage if undertaken within a few hours of ingestion. Very large dosage may depress central nervous system. There is no specific antidote and treatment is supportive.

ETHAMBUTOL

It is a synthetic congener of 1, 2-ethanediamine. It is a bacteriostatic drug.

Mechanism of Action

It interferes with mycolic acid incorporation in cell wall and has been shown to inhibit RNA synthesis. Bacterial resistance to drug develops in vivo via single amino acid change in embA genes when given in absence of another effective agent.

Distribution

It is widely distributed but penetrates meninges incompletely.

Excretion

It is excreted in urine by glomerular filtration and tubular secretion.

Preparation and Dose

Ethambutol is supplied in 400 mg, 600 mg, 800 mg and 1000 mg tablets. Combined preparations with isoniazid are available.

The dosage for daily therapy being 15 (15–20) mg/kg/day and in twice weekly regimen dosage is 45 (40–50) /mg/kg/day and in thrice weekly regimen dosage is 30 (25–35) mg/kg/day.

Pregnancy

Ethambutol is safer in pregnancy.

Side Effects

Common side effects include retrobulbar optic neuritis and hyperuricemia. Rare side effects include fever, rash, hypersensitivity reaction, gastrointestinal upset, neurological disturbances (dizziness, confusion and hallucinations), thrombocytopenia.

Renal Disease

There is significant renal excretion of ethambutol and hence dose adjustment is required in patients with renal insufficiency.

Contraindications

Ethambutol is contraindicated in patients with known hypersensitivity, previously existing visual disorder and renal failure.

Overdosage

Overdosage of ethambutol can be reverted by induced emesis and gastric lavage if undertaken within a few hours of ingestion. Subsequently, dialysis may be of value. There is no specific antidote and treatment is supportive.

PYRAZINAMIDE

It is a synthetic pyrazine analogue of nicotinamide. It is a bactericidal drug. It is more active in acidic medium. Hence, it acts on intracellular bacilli as well as on bacilli at sites of inflammatory response.

Mechanism of Action

It inhibits mycobacterial mycolic acid synthesis by acting on mycobacterial fatty acid synthase I gene.

Distribution

It is widely distributed in body and has good penetration in CSF.

Excretion

It is extensively metabolized in liver and excreted in urine.

Preparation and Dose

The drug is available in 500 mg, 1,000 mg and 1,500 mg or combined preparation with rifampicin plus isoniazid. The dose for daily patients being 25 (20–30) mg/kg and in twice weekly regimen dosage is 50 (40–60)/mg/kg/day and in thrice weekly regimen dosage is 35 (30–40) mg/kg/day.

Pregnancy

Pyrazinamide is safer in pregnancy.

Side Effects

Common side effects include hepatitis and hyperuricemia. Rare side effects include fever, rashes, loss of diabetes control and gastrointestinal upset and thrombocytopenia.

Renal Disease

There is significant renal excretion of metabolites of pyrazinamide and hence dose adjustment is required in patients with renal insufficiency.

Contraindications

Pyrazinamide is contraindicated in known hypersensitivity and hepatic dysfunction.

Overdosage

Overdosage of pyrazinamide may result in acute liver damage and hyperuricemia. It is reverted by gastric lavage and induced emesis if undertaken within a few hours of ingestion. There is no specific antidote.

STREPTOMYCIN

It is an aminoglycoside antibiotic derived from *Streptomyces griseus*. It is bactericidal drug. It acts only on extracellular bacilli.

Mechanism of Action

Streptomycin binds to several sites at 30S and 50S subunits of the ribosome as well as to their interface thereby interfering with polysome formation and causing misreading of mRNA code.

Distribution

It penetrates tubercular cavities but it does not penetrate cell walls or normal biological membranes such as the meninges or the pleura unless inflammatory changes have taken place. It crosses the placenta and fetal serum levels are about half those in maternal blood.

Excretion

It is excreted unchanged in the urine mainly by glomerular filtration.

Preparation and Dose

Streptomycin sulfate for intramuscular injection is supplied as a powder in vials and should be reconstituted immediately before use. The dose for daily therapy being 15 (range 12–18) mg/kg/day and same in twice or thrice weekly regimen. Patients aged over 60 years may not be able to tolerate more than 500–750 mg daily.

Side Effects

Common side effects are pain at site of injection, auditory ototoxicity, vestibular toxicity and nephrotoxicity. Rare side effects include hemolytic anemia, agranulocytosis, thrombocytopenia and hypersensitivity reaction.

Renal Disease

Because of an increased risk of nephrotoxicity and ototoxicity, streptomycin should be avoided in patients with renal failure.

Pregnancy

It should not be given in pregnancy as it crosses the placental barrier producing ototoxicity (auditory nerve impairment) and renal impairment in the fetus.

Contraindications

It should not be given in known hypersensitivity, auditory nerve impairment, myasthenia gravis and renal failure.

Overdosage

In case of overdosage of streptomycin, hemodialysis may be beneficial. There is no specific antidote and treatment is supportive.

FURTHER READINGS

1. Byrd RB, Horn. BR, Solomon DA, Griggs GA. Toxic effects of isoniazid in tuberculosis chemoprophylaxis. Role of biochemical monitoring in 1000 patients. JAMA. 1979;241;1239–41.
2. Garg R, Gupta V, Mehra S, Singh R, Prasad R. Rifampicin induced thrombocytopenia. Indian J Tub. 2007;54:94-6.
3. Garg R, Vaibhav, Mehra S, Prasad R. Isoniazid induced gynaecomastia: a case report. Indian J Tuberculosis. 2009;56:51-4.
4. Jhonston RN, et al. Prolonged streptomycin and isoniazid for pulmonary tuberculosis. BMJ. 1964;1:1679-83.
5. Kant S, Verma SK, Gupta V, Anand SC, Prasad R. Pyrazinamide induced thrombocytopenia. Indian J Pharmacol. 2010;42:108-9.
6. Peloquin CA, et al. Pharmacokinetics of isoniazid under fasting condition, with food and antacids. Int J Tub and Lung Dis. 1999;3:703-10.
7. Prasad R, Garg R, Verma SK. Isoniazid- and ethambutol-induced psychosis. Annals of Thoracic Med. 2008;3:149-51.
8. Prasad R, Mukherji PK. Ethambutol induced thrombocytopenia. Tubercle. 1989;70:211-2.
9. Prasad R, Mukherji PK. Rifampicin induced thrombocytopenia. Ind J Tub. 1989;36:44-5.
10. Steele MA, Burk RF, DesPrez RM. Toxic hepatitis with isoniazid and rifampicin: a meta analysis. Chest. 1991;99:465-71.

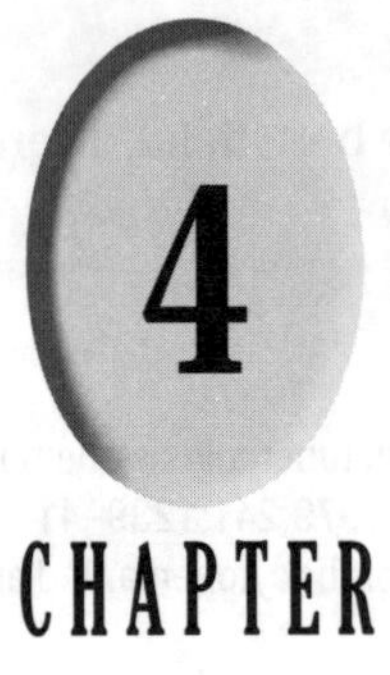

CHAPTER 4 Pharmacology of Antitubercular Drugs Used in Drug Resistant Patients of Tuberculosis

KANAMYCIN

Drug Class

Aminoglycoside

Activity against TB, Mechanism of Action and Metabolism

Bactericidal, aminoglycosides inhibit protein synthesis by irreversibly binding to 30 S ribosomal subunit; aminoglycosides are not metabolized in the liver, they are excreted unchanged in the urine.

Distribution

0.2–0.4 L/kg; distributed in extracellular fluid, abscesses, ascitic fluid, pericardial fluid, pleural fluid, synovial fluid, lymphatic fluid and peritoneal fluid. Not well distributed into bile, aqueous humor, bronchial secretions, sputum and cerebrospinal fluid (CSF).

Preparation and Dose

Kanamycin sulfate, sterile powder for intramuscular injection in sealed vials. The powder needs to be dissolved in water for injections before use. The optimal dose is 15 mg/kg body weight, usually 750 mg to 1 g given daily or 5–6 days per week, by deep intramuscular injection. Rotation of injection sites avoids local discomfort. When necessary, it is possible to give the drug at the same total dose 2 or 3 times weekly during the continuation phase, under close monitoring for adverse effects.

Storage

Powder stable at room temperature (15°–25°C), diluted solution should be used the same day.

Oral Absorption

There is no significant oral absorption.

CSF Penetration

Penetrates inflamed meninges only.

Special Circumstances

Pregnancy/breastfeeding

Safety class D. Eighth cranial nerve damage has been reported following in utero exposure to kanamycin. Excreted in breast milk. The American Academy of Pediatrics (AAP) considers kanamycin to be compatible with breastfeeding.

Renal Disease

Use with caution. Levels should be monitored for patients with impaired renal function. Interval adjustment (12–15 mg/kg 2 or 3 times per week) is recommended for creatinine clearance < 30 mL/minute or hemodialysis.

Hepatic Disease

Drug levels not affected by hepatic disease (except a larger volume of distribution for alcoholic cirrhotic patients with ascites). Presumed to be safe in severe liver disease; however, use with caution as some patients with severe liver disease may progress rapidly to hepatorenal syndrome.

Adverse Effects

Frequent

- Pain at injection site
- Renal failure (usually reversible).

Occasional

- Vestibular and auditory damage (usually irreversible)
- Nephrotoxicity (dose-related to cumulative and peak concentrations)
- Increased risk with renal insufficiency (often irreversible)
- Peripheral neuropathy
- Rash.

Ototoxicity potentiated by certain diuretics (especially loop diuretics), advanced age, and prolonged use. The effect of nondepolarizing muscle relaxants may be increased.

Contraindications

- Pregnancy (congenital deafness seen with streptomycin and kanamycin use in pregnancy)
- Hypersensitivity to aminoglycosides
- Caution with renal, hepatic, vestibular or auditory impairment.

Monitoring

Monthly creatinine and serum potassium in low-risk patients (young with no comorbidities), more frequently in high-risk patients (elderly, diabetic, or HIV-positive patients, or patients with renal insufficiency). If potassium is low, check magnesium and calcium. Baseline audiometry and monthly monitoring in high-risk patients. For problems with balance, consider increasing dosing interval.

Alerting Symptoms

- Problems with hearing
- Dizziness
- Rash
- Trouble breathing
- Decreased urination
- Swelling, pain or redness at injection site
- Muscle twitching or weakness.

AMIKACIN

Drug Class

Aminoglycoside

Activity against TB, Mechanism of Action and Metabolism

Bactericidal, inhibit protein synthesis through disruption of ribosomal function; less effective in acidic pH, aminoglycosides are not metabolized in the liver, they are excreted unchanged in the urine.

Preparation and Dose

Amikacin sulfate, colorless solution. 250 mg/mL (2 or 4 mL vials) and 50 mg/mL (2 mL vial). The optimal dose is 15–20 mg/kg body weight, usually 750 mg to 1 g given daily or 5–6 days per week by deep intramuscular injection. Rotation of injection sites avoids local discomfort. When necessary, it is possible to give the drug at the same total dose 2 or 3 times weekly during the continuation phase under close monitoring for adverse effects.

Storage

Solution is stable at room temperature (15°–25°C); diluted solution is stable at room temperature for at least 3 days or in the refrigerator for at least 60 days.

Oral Absorption

There is no significant oral absorption. Intramuscular absorption may be delayed if the same site is used consistently.

CSF Penetration

Penetrates inflamed meninges only.

Special Circumstances

Pregnancy/breastfeeding

Safety class D. No reports linking the use of amikacin to congenital defects have been reported. Ototoxicity has not been reported as an effect of in utero exposure to amikacin; however, eighth cranial nerve toxicity in the fetus is well known following exposure to other aminoglycosides (kanamycin and streptomycin) and could potentially occur with amikacin. Only a trace amount of amikacin was found in some nursing infants. Given the poor absorption of aminoglycosides, systemic toxicity should not occur, but alteration in normal bowel flora may occur in nursing infants.

Renal Disease

Use with caution. Levels should be monitored for patients with impaired renal function. Interval adjustment (12–15 mg/kg 2 or 3 times per week) is recommended for creatinine clearance < 30 mL/min or hemodialysis.

Hepatic Disease

Drug levels not affected by hepatic disease (except a larger volume of distribution for alcoholic cirrhotic patients with ascites). Presumed to be safe in severe liver disease; however, some patients with severe liver disease may progress rapidly to hepatorenal syndrome.

Adverse Effects

Frequent

- Pain at injection site
- Proteinuria
- Serum electrolyte disturbances including hypokalemia and hypomagnesemia.

Occasional

- Cochlear ototoxicity (may be irreversible)
- Nephrotoxicity (often irreversible)
- Peripheral neuropathy
- Rash
- Vestibular toxicity (nausea, vomiting, vertigo, ataxia, nystagmus)
- Eosinophilia

Ototoxicity potentiated by certain diuretics (especially loop diuretics), advanced age, and prolonged use. The effect of nondepolarizing muscle relaxants may be increased.

Contraindications

- Pregnancy (congenital deafness seen with streptomycin and kanamycin use in pregnancy)
- Hypersensitivity to aminoglycosides
- Caution with renal, hepatic, vestibular, or auditory impairment.

Monitoring

Monthly creatinine and serum potassium in low-risk patients (young with no comorbidities), more frequently in high-risk patients (elderly, diabetic, or HIV-positive patients, or patients with renal insufficiency). If potassium is low, check magnesium and calcium. Baseline audiometry and monthly monitoring in high-risk patients. For problems with balance, consider increasing dosing interval.

Alerting Symptoms

- Problems with hearing, dizziness or balance
- Rash or swelling of the face
- Trouble breathing
- Decreased urination
- Swelling, pain or redness at IM site
- Muscle twitching or weakness.

CAPREOMYCIN

Drug Class

Cyclic polypeptide

Activity against TB, Mechanism of Action and Metabolism

Bactericidal, Polypeptides appear to inhibit translocation of the peptidyl-tRNA and the initiation of protein synthesis. No cross-resistance with the aminoglycosides. 50–60% excreted via glomerulofiltration. Small amount by biliary excretion.

Preparation and Dose

Capreomycin sulfate is supplied as a sterile white powder for intramuscular injection in sealed vials each containing 1,000 units, approximately equivalent to 1 g capreomycin base. This should be dissolved in 2 mL of 0.9% sodium chloride in water; 2–3 minutes should be allowed for complete solution. Dose: 15–20 mg/kg daily. The usual dose is 1 g in a single dose daily. When necessary, it is possible to give the drug at the same dose 2 or 3 times weekly during the continuation phase, under close monitoring for adverse effects.

Storage

Reconstituted capreomycin can be stored in the refrigerator for up to 24 hours before use.

Oral Absorption

There is no significant oral absorption. Intramuscular absorption may be delayed if the same site is used consistently.

CSF Penetration

Penetrates inflamed meninges only.

Special Circumstances

Pregnancy/breastfeeding

Less ototoxicity reported in adults with capreomycin than with aminoglycosides. Category C animal studies show teratogenic effect ("wavy ribs" when given 3.5 times the human dose). Avoid in pregnancy. Concentrations in breast milk unknown.

Renal Disease

Use with caution. Levels should be monitored for patients with impaired renal function. Interval adjustment (12–15 mg/kg 2 or 3 times per week) is recommended for creatinine clearance < 30 mL/min or hemodialysis.

Adverse Effects

Frequent

- Nephrotoxicity (20–25%)
- Tubular dysfunction
- Azotemia, proteinuria
- Urticaria or maculopapular rash.

Occasional

- Ototoxicity (vestibular > auditory)
- Electrolyte abnormalities (decreased blood levels of calcium, magnesium, and potassium)
- Pain, induration and sterile abscesses at injection sites.

Contraindications

Patients with hypersensitivity to capreomycin. Great caution must be exercised in patients with renal insufficiency or pre-existing auditory impairment.

Monitoring

Monthly creatinine and serum potassium in low-risk patients (young with no comorbidities), more frequently in high-risk patients (elderly, diabetic, or HIV-positive patients, or patients with renal insufficiency). If potassium is low, check magnesium and calcium. Electrolyte disturbances are more common with capreomycin than other injectable agents. Baseline audiometry and monthly monitoring in high-risk patients. For problems with balance, consider increasing dosing interval.

Alerting Symptoms

- Rash
- Decreased urination
- Fever or chills
- Trouble breathing
- Bleeding or bruising
- Muscle weakness
- Problems with hearing, dizziness or balance
- Bleeding or lump at intramuscular injection site.

CYCLOSERINE/TERIZIDONE

Drug Class

Analog of D-alanine

Activity against TB, Mechanism of Action and Metabolism

Bacteriostatic, competitively blocks the enzyme that incorporates alanine into an alanyl-alanine dipeptide, an essential component of the mycobacterial cell wall. No cross-resistance with other antituberculosis drugs. 60–70% excreted unchanged in the urine via glomerular filtration; small amount excreted in feces; small amount metabolized.

Preparation and Dose

Capsules (250 mg). 10–15 mg/kg daily (maximum 1,000 mg), usually 500–750 mg per day given in two divided doses (Some producers of terizidone make 300 mg capsule preparations, while others make 250 mg).

Storage

Room temperature (15°–25°C) in airtight containers.

Oral Absorption

Modestly decreased by food (best to take on an empty stomach); 70–90% absorbed.

Distribution

Widely distributed into body tissue and fluids such as lung, bile, ascitic fluid, pleural fluid, synovial fluid, lymph, sputum. Very good CSF penetration (80–100% of serum concentration attained in the CSF, higher level with inflamed meninges).

Special Circumstances

Pregnancy/breastfeeding

Safety class C. Breastfeeding with B6 supplement to the infant.

Renal Disease

Doses of cycloserine should be reduced in patients with severe renal impairment. When the creatinine clearance is less than 30 mL/min, the recommended dosing is 250 mg/day, or 500 mg/dose 3 times per week. The appropriateness of 250 mg/day doses has not been established. There should be careful monitoring for evidence of neurotoxicity; if possible, measure serum concentrations and adjust regimen accordingly.

Adverse Effects

Frequent

- Neurological and psychiatric disturbances (headaches, irritability, sleep disturbances, aggression, and tremors)
- Gum inflammation
- Pale skin
- Depression, confusion, dizziness, restlessness, anxiety, nightmares, severe headache, drowsiness.

Occasional

- Visual changes
- Skin rash
- Numbness, tingling or burning in hands and feet
- Jaundice
- Eye pain.

Rare

Seizures, suicidal thoughts.

Contraindications

Hypersensitivity to cycloserine, epilepsy, depression, severe anxiety or psychosis, severe renal insufficiency, excessive concurrent use of alcohol.

Monitoring

When available, serum drug monitoring to establish optimal dosing (not higher than 30 μg/mL).

Alerting Symptoms

- Seizures
- Shakiness or trouble talking
- Depression or thoughts of intentional self-harm
- Anxiety, confusion or loss of memory
- Personality changes, such as aggressive behavior
- Rash or hives
- Headache.

ETHIONAMIDE AND PROTHIONAMIDE

Drug Class

Carbothionamides group, derivatives of isonicotinic acid.

Activity against TB, Mechanism of Action and Metabolism

Bacteriostatic, the mechanism of action of thionamides has not been fully elucidated, but they appear to inhibit mycolic acid synthesis. Resistance develops rapidly if used alone and there is complete cross-resistance between ethionamide and prothionamide (partial cross-resistance with thioacetazone). Ethionamide is extensively metabolized, probably in the liver, to the active sulfoxide and other inactive metabolites and less than 1% of a dose appears in the urine as unchanged drug.

Preparation and Dose

Ethionamide and prothionamide are normally administered in the form of tablets containing 125 mg or 250 mg of active drug. The maximum optimum daily dose is 15–20 mg/kg/day (maximum 1 g/day), usually 500–750 mg.

Storage

Room temperature (15°–25°C) in airtight containers.

Oral Absorption

About 100% absorbed but sometimes erratic absorption caused by gastrointestinal disturbances associated with the medication.

Distribution

Rapidly and widely distributed into body tissues and fluids, with concentrations in plasma and various organs being approximately equal. Significant concentrations also are present in CSF.

Special Circumstances

Pregnancy/breastfeeding

Safety class C. Animal studies have shown ethionamide to be teratogenic. Newborns who are breastfed by mothers who are taking ethionamide should be monitored for adverse effects.

Renal Disease

Doses of the thionamides are only slightly modified for patients with severe renal impairment. When the creatinine clearance is less than 30 mL/minute, the recommended dosing is 250–500 mg daily.

Hepatic Disease

Thionamides should not be used in severe hepatic impairment.

Porphyria

Ethionamide is considered to be unsafe in patients with porphyria because it has been shown to be porphyrinogenic in animals and in vitro systems.

Adverse Effects

Frequent

Severe gastrointestinal intolerance (nausea, vomiting, diarrhea, abdominal pain, excessive salivation, metallic taste, stomatitis, anorexia and weight loss). Adverse gastrointestinal effects appear to be dose-related, with approximately 50% of patients unable to tolerate 1 g as a single dose. Gastrointestinal effects may be minimized by decreasing dosage, by changing the time of drug administration, or by the concurrent administration of an antiemetic agent.

Occasional

Allergic reactions, psychotic disturbances (including depression), drowsiness, dizziness, restlessness, headache, postural hypotension, neurotoxicity (administration of pyridoxine has been recommended to prevent or relieve neurotoxic effects), transient increases in serum bilirubin; reversible hepatitis (2%) with jaundice (1–3%), gynecomastia; menstrual irregularity, arthralgias, leukopenia, hypothyroidism especially when combined with para-aminosalicylic acid (PAS).

Rare

Peripheral neuritis, optic neuritis, diplopia, blurred vision, pellagra-like syndrome, reactions including rash, photosensitivity, thrombocytopenia and purpura.

Contraindications

Thionamides are contraindicated in patients with severe hepatic impairment and in patients who are hypersensitive to these drugs.

Monitoring

Ophthalmological examinations should be performed before and periodically during therapy. Periodic monitoring of blood glucose and thyroid function is desirable. Diabetic patients should be particularly alert for episodes of hypoglycemia. Liver function tests should be carried out before and during treatment with ethionamide.

Alerting Symptoms

- Any problems with eyes: Eye pain, blurred vision, color blindness, or trouble seeing
- Numbness, tingling, or pain in hands and feet
- Unusual bruising or bleeding
- Personality changes such as depression, confusion or aggression
- Yellowing of skin
- Dark-colored urine
- Nausea and vomiting
- Dizziness.

PARA-AMINOSALICYLIC ACID (PAS)

Drug Class

Salicylic acid; antifolate

Activity against TB, Mechanism of Action and Metabolism

Bacteriostatic, disrupts folic acid metabolism. Acetylated in the liver to *N*-acetyl-para-aminosalicylic acid and para-aminosalicylic acid, which are excreted via glomerular filtration and tubular secretion.

Preparation and Dose

Tablets, sugar-coated, containing sodium salt: Sodium para-aminosalicylate, 0.5 g of PAS. Granules of PAS with an acid-resistant outer coating rapidly dissolved in neutral media, 4 g per packet.
150 mg/kg or 10–12 g daily in 2 divided doses.
Children: 200–300 mg/kg daily in 2–4 divided doses.

Storage

Packets should be kept in the refrigerator or freezer. Other formulations may not require refrigeration (consult manufacturer's recommendations).

Oral Absorption

Incomplete absorption (usually 60–65%): Sometimes requires increased doses to achieve therapeutic levels.

Distribution

Distributed in peritoneal fluid, pleural fluid, synovial fluid. Not well distributed in CSF (10–15%) and bile.

Special Circumstances

Pregnancy/breastfeeding

Safety class C. Congenital defects in babies have been reported with exposure to PAS in the first trimester. PAS is secreted into human breast milk (1/70th of maternal plasma concentration).

Renal Disease

No dose adjustment is recommended. However, PAS can exacerbate acidosis associated with renal insufficiency and if possible should be avoided in patients with severe renal impairment due to crystalluria. Sodium PAS should also be avoided in patients with severe renal impairment.

Adverse Effects

Frequent

- Gastrointestinal intolerance (anorexia and diarrhea)
- Hypothyroidism (increased risk with concomitant use of ethionamide).

Occasional

- Hepatitis (0.3–0.5%)
- Allergic reactions
- Thyroid enlargement
- Malabsorption syndrome
- Increased prothrombin time
- Fever.

Careful use in patients with glucose-6-phosphate dehydrogenase (G6PD) deficiency.

Contraindications

Allergy to aspirin; severe renal disease; hypersensitivity to the drug.

Monitoring

Monitor TSH, electrolytes, blood counts and liver function tests.

Alerting Symptoms

- Skin rash, severe itching, or hives
- Severe abdominal pain, nausea or vomiting
- Unusual tiredness or loss of appetite
- Black stools as a result of intestinal bleeding.

LEVOFLOXACIN

Drug Class

Fluoroquinolone

Activity against TB, Mechanism of Action and Metabolism

Bactericidal, acts by inhibiting the A subunit of DNA gyrase (topoisomerase), which is essential in the reproduction of bacterial DNA. Levofloxacin is generally considered to be about twice as active as its isomer, ofloxacin. Minimal hepatic metabolism; 87% of dose excreted unchanged in the urine within 48 hours via glomerular filtration and tubular secretion.

Preparation and Dose

Tablets (250, 500, 750 mg). Aqueous solution or solution in 5% dextrose for IV administration—vials (20, 30 mL) 500 or 750 mg and flexible containers (50,100, 150 mL) 250; 500 or 750 mg.
Usual dose: 750 mg/day.

Storage

Tablets: Room temperature (15°–25°C), airtight containers protected from light.

Oral Absorption

Levofloxacin is rapidly and essentially completely absorbed after oral administration. Orally, should not be administered within 4 hours of other medications containing divalent cations (iron, magnesium, zinc, vitamins, didanosine, sucralfate). No interaction with milk or calcium.

Distribution

Distributes well in blister fluid and lung tissues, also widely distributed (kidneys, gallbladder, gynecological tissues, liver, lung, prostatic tissue, phagocytic cells, urine, sputum and bile). 30–50% of serum concentration is attained in CSF with inflamed meninges.

Special Circumstances

Pregnancy/breastfeeding

Safety class C. There are no adequate and well-controlled studies in pregnant women. Levofloxacin should be used during pregnancy only if the potential benefit justifies the potential risk to the fetus. Animal data demonstrated arthropathy in immature animals, with erosions in joint cartilage. Because of the potential for serious adverse effects from levofloxacin in nursing infants, a decision should be made whether to discontinue nursing or to discontinue the drug, taking into account the importance of the drug to the mother.

Renal Disease

Doses of levofloxacin should be reduced in patients with severe renal impairment. When the creatinine clearance is less than 30 mL/min, the recommended dosing is 750–1,000 mg 3 times per week.

Hepatic Disease

Given the limited extent of levofloxacin metabolism, the pharmacokinetics of levofloxacin are not expected to be affected by hepatic impairment.

Adverse Effects

Generally well tolerated.

Occasional

- Gastrointestinal intolerance
- Central nervous system (CNS)—headache; malaise; insomnia; restlessness; dizziness
- Allergic reactions
- Diarrhea
- Photosensitivity.

Rare

- QT prolongation
- Tendon rupture
- Peripheral neuropathy.

Contraindications

- Pregnancy
- Hypersensitivity to fluoroquinolones
- Prolonged QT interval.

Monitoring

No specific laboratory monitoring requirements.

Alerting Symptoms

- Pain, swelling or tearing of a tendon or muscle or joint pain
- Rashes, hives, bruising or blistering, trouble breathing
- Diarrhea
- Yellow skin or eyes
- Anxiety, confusion or dizziness.

MOXIFLOXACIN

Drug Class

Fluoroquinolone

Activity against TB, Mechanism of Action and Metabolism

Bactericidal, acts by inhibiting the A subunit of DNA gyrase (topoisomerase), which is essential in the reproduction of bacterial DNA. The cytochrome P450 system is not involved in moxifloxacin metabolism, and is not affected by moxifloxacin. Approximately 45% of an oral or intravenous dose of moxifloxacin is excreted as unchanged drug (~20% in urine and ~25% in feces). Preparation and dose tablets 400 mg and intravenous solution 250 mL–400 mg in 0.8% saline. Usual dose: 400 mg/day.

Storage

Tablets: Room temperature (15°–25°C), airtight containers protected from light.

Oral Absorption

Moxifloxacin, given as an oral tablet, is well absorbed from the gastrointestinal tract. The absolute bioavailability of moxifloxacin is approximately 90%. Co-administration with a high fat meal (e.g. 500 calories from fat) does not affect the absorption of moxifloxacin.

Distribution

Moxifloxacin has been detected in the saliva, nasal and bronchial secretions, mucosa of the sinuses, skin blister fluid, and subcutaneous tissue, and skeletal muscle following oral or intravenous administration of 400 mg.

Special Circumstances

Pregnancy/breastfeeding

Safety class C. Since there are no adequate or well-controlled studies in pregnant women, moxifloxacin should be used during pregnancy only if the potential benefit justifies the potential risk to the fetus. Because of the potential for serious adverse effects in infants nursing from mothers taking moxifloxacin, a decision should be made whether to discontinue nursing or to discontinue the drug, taking into account the importance of the drug to the mother.

Renal Disease

No dosage adjustment is required in renally impaired patients, including those on either hemodialysis or continuous ambulatory peritoneal dialysis.

Hepatic Disease

No dosage adjustment is required in patients with mild or moderate hepatic insufficiency.

Adverse Effects

Generally well tolerated.

Occasional

- Gastrointestinal intolerance, CNS—headache; malaise; insomnia; restlessness; dizziness
- Allergic reactions
- Diarrhea
- Photosensitivity
- QT prolongation
- Tendon rupture
- Photosensitivity
- Moxifloxacin has been found in isolated cases to prolong the QT interval.

Contraindications

- Pregnancy
- Hypersensitivity to fluoroquinolones
- Prolonged QT interval.

Monitoring

No specific laboratory monitoring requirements.

Alerting Symptoms

- Pain, swelling or tearing of a tendon or muscle or joint pain
- Rashes, hives, bruising or blistering, trouble breathing
- Diarrhea
- Yellow skin or eyes
- Anxiety, confusion or dizziness.

OFLOXACIN

Drug Class

Fluoroquinolones

Activity against TB, Mechanism of Action and Metabolism

Bactericidal, acts by inhibiting the A subunit of DNA gyrase (topoisomerase), which is essential in the reproduction of bacterial DNA. There is no cross-resistance with other antituberculosis agents, but complete cross-resistance between ofloxacin and ciprofloxacin. There is limited metabolism to desmethyl and N-oxide metabolites; desmethylofloxacin has moderate antibacterial activity.

Ofloxacin is eliminated mainly by the kidneys. Excretion is by tubular secretion and glomerular filtration and 65–80% of a dose is excreted unchanged in the urine over 24–48 hours, resulting in high urinary concentrations.

Preparation and Dose

Tablets (200, 300 or 400 mg). Vials (10 mL) or flexible containers (50 and 100 mL) with aqueous or 5% dextrose IV solutions equivalent to 200 and 400 mg. Usual dose: 400 mg twice daily.

Storage

Room temperature (15°–25°C), airtight containers protected from light.

Oral Absorption

90–98% oral absorption.

Distribution

About 25% is bound to plasma proteins. Ofloxacin is widely distributed in body fluids, including the CSF, and tissue penetration is good. It crosses the placenta and is distributed into breast milk. It also appears in the bile.

Special Circumstances

Pregnancy/breastfeeding

Usually compatible with breastfeeding.

Renal Disease

Doses of ofloxacin should be reduced in patients with severe renal impairment. When the creatinine clearance is less than 30 mL/min, the recommended dosing is 600–800 mg 3 times per week.

Adverse Effects

Generally well tolerated.

Occasional

- Gastrointestinal intolerance
- CNS—headache, malaise, insomnia, restlessness, and dizziness.

Rare

- Allergic reactions
- Diarrhea
- Photosensitivity
- Increased liver function tests (LFTs)

- Tendon rupture
- Peripheral neuropathy.

Contraindications

Pregnancy, intolerance of fluoroquinolones.

Monitoring

No specific laboratory monitoring requirements.

Alerting Symptoms

- Pain, swelling or tearing of a tendon or muscle or joint pain
- Rashes, hives, bruising or blistering, trouble breathing
- Diarrhea
- Yellow skin or eyes
- Anxiety, confusion or dizziness

GATIFLOXACIN

Drug Class

Fluoroquinolone

Activity against TB, Mechanism of Action and Metabolism

Bactericidal: Acts by inhibiting the A subunit of DNA gyrase (topoisomerase), which is essential in the reproduction of and metabolism bacterial DNA.

Preparation and Dose

Tablets— 200 or 400 mg.
Dose— 400 mg/day.

Storage

Room temperature (15–25 °C), airtight containers protected from light.

Oral Absorption

Readily absorbed from the gastrointestinal tract with an absolute bioavailability of 96%. Gatifloxacin in an anion and taking with divalent cations will result in bonding and not being absorbed. Administrate two hours before or four hours after ingestion of milk-based products, antacids or other medications containing divalent cations (iron, magnesium, calcium, zinc, vitamins, didanosine, sucralfate).

CSF Penetration

Widely distributed in body fluids including CSF.

Special Circumstances

Pregnancy/breastfeeding

Safety class C. Fluoroquinolones are not recommended during breastfeeding due to the potential for arthropathy. Animal data demonstrated arthropathy in immature animals, with erosions in joint cartilage.

Renal Disease

Doses of gatifloxacin should be reduced in patients with renal impairment. when creatinine clearance is less than 30 mL/min, the recommended dosing is 400 mg, 3 times per week.

Adverse Effects

Generally well tolerated.

Occasional

Gastrointestinal intolerance.

Rare

- CNS—headache
- Malaise
- Insomnia
- Restlessness
- Dizziness
- Allergic reactions
- Diarrhea
- Photosensitivity
- Increased liver function tests
- Tendon rupture (increased incidence seen in older men with concurrent use of corticosteroids)
- Severe dysglycemia, hypoglycemia and hyperglycemia, and diabetes have been reported (many countries have removed the drug form their national formularies for this reason).

Contraindications

- Pregnancy
- Intolerance of fluoroquinolones
- Diabetes. Gatifloxacin can worsen diabetes and glycemic control.

Monitoring

Glucose monitoring every 1–2 weeks.

Alerting Symptoms

- Rashes, hives, bruising or blistering, trouble breathing

- Pain, swelling or tearing of a tendon or muscle or joint pain.
- Diarrhea
- Yellow skin or eyes
- Anxiety, confusion or dizziness (signs of hypoglycemia or hyperglycemia)
- Increased thirst or frequent urination (sign of hyperglycemia).

CLOFAZIMINE

Drug Class

Phenazine derivative

Activity against TB, Mechanism of Action and Metabolism

Bacteriostatic against *M. leprae*, active in vitro against *M. tuberculosis*. Clinical effectiveness against *M. tuberculosis* not well established. Clofazimine appears to bind preferentially to mycobacterial DNA (principally at base sequences containing guanine) and inhibit mycobacterial replication and growth. Excreted in feces as unabsorbed drug and via biliary elimination. Little urinary excretion.

Preparation and Dose

Capsules (50 and 100 mg).
Dose: Adults: 100–200 mg daily (oral) has been used. A regimen of 200 mg daily for 2 months, followed by 100 mg daily has been used.
Children: Limited data, but doses of 1 mg/kg/day.

Storage

Store below 30°C, in airtight containers.

Oral Absorption

About 20–70% absorbed from gastrointestinal tract.

Distribution

Widely distributed principally to fatty tissue, reticuloendothelial system and macrophages. High concentrations found in mesenteric lymph nodes, adipose tissue, adrenals, liver, lungs, in gallbladder, bile and spleen.

Special Circumstances

Pregnancy/breastfeeding

Safety class C. Animal studies demonstrated teratogenicity (retardation of fetal skull ossification). Crosses placenta and is excreted in milk. Not recommended during breastfeeding.

Renal Disease

Usual dose.

Hepatic Disease

Dose adjustments should be considered in patients with severe hepatic insufficiency.

Adverse Effects

Frequent

- Ichthyosis and dry skin
- Pink to brownish-black discoloration of skin, cornea, retina and urine
- Anorexia
- Abdominal pain.

Contraindications

- Pregnancy
- Severe hepatic insufficiency
- Hypersensitivity to clofazimine.

Monitoring

No specific laboratory monitoring requirements.

Alerting Symptoms

- Bloody or black stools or diarrhoea
- Yellowing of skin or eyes
- Severe nausea, vomiting, abdominal pain, cramps or burning
- Depression or thoughts of hurting one-self.

THIACETAZONE

Drug Class

Thiosemicarbazone. It is a bacteriostatic drug of low efficacy. It delays resistance to other anti-tubercular drugs like streptomycin, isoniazid and ethambutol.

Pharmacokinetics

It is orally active and primarily excreted unchanged in urine.

Preparation and Dose

The daily dosage recommended is 2.5 mg/kg body weight daily; it is not effective when given intermittently.

Contraindications

In HIV positive patients, the risk of major potentially fatal cutaneous reaction caused by thioacetazone is very high. It should never be used in patients who may be HIV-positive or in areas where HIV infection is common.

Adverse Effects

Frequent

- Gastrointestinal intolerance
- Rash
- Anemia.

Occasional

- Hepatitis
- Exfoliative dermatitis and Stevens-Johnson syndrome.

Rare

- Bone marrow depression
- Ototoxicity.

Special Circumstances

Renal Disease

It should be avoided when renal impairment is present.

Pregnancy/Breastfeeding

Studies on the effects of thiacetazone in pregnancy and breastfeeding have not been done in humans or animals.

Monitoring

No specific laboratory monitoring requirements.

RIFABUTIN

Drug Class

Rifamycin

Activity against TB, Mechanism of Action and Metabolism

Bactericidal, same mechanism of activity as rifampin (inhibits RNA polymerase). Less than 20% of rifampin-resistant strains are susceptible to rifabutin.

Preparation and Dose

150 mg capsule

Dose: Adults: 5 mg/kg/dose (max dose 300 mg, though doses up to 450 mg are sometimes used). Dose adjustments sometimes required when dosing with interacting drugs.

Children: The pediatric dose is not established, but doses of 5–10 mg/kg/day have been used (higher doses have been recommended for children <1 year of age). Caution is advised when used in very young children in whom visual changes might not be obvious.

Storage

Capsules should be kept at room temperature (15–25 °C).

Oral Absorption

Well absorbed from the gastrointestinal tract.

CSF Penetration

Penetrates inflamed meninges.

Special Circumstances

Pregnancy/breastfeeding

Insufficient data about use during pregnancy. Unknown effects from breastfeeding.

Renal Disease

Used without dose adjustment in mild renal insufficiency. For creatinine clearance <30 mL/minute, the usual dose may be used, but monitor drug concentrations to avoid toxicity.

Hepatic Disease

Use with caution and additional monitoring in liver disease.

Adverse Effects

- Leukopenia (dose dependent); thrombocytopenia
- Rashes and skin discoloration (bronzing or pseudojaundice)
- Anterior uveitis and other eye toxicities
- Hepatotoxicity similar to that of rifampin
- Arthralgias
- Drug interactions with many other drugs—but only 40% of that is seen with rifampin. Rifabutin concentrations may be affected by other drugs.

Contraindications

Rifamycin hypersensitivity. Data are lacking on cross-sensitivity to rifabutin in patients with hypersensitivity. If used, use with caution, with careful monitoring of patient for development of hypersensitivity. Should not be used for patients with MDR-TB.

Monitoring

Increased liver function monitoring; monitor drug concentrations of interacting medications; blood counts and vision screening.

Alerting Symptoms

- Any eye pain, change in vision or sensitivity to light
- Fever, chills or sore throat
- Pain or swelling in the joints
- Yellowing of the skin or eyes or dark urine
- Nausea or vomiting
- Unusual tiredness or loss of appetite.

RIFAPENTINE

Drug Class

Rifamycin

Activity against TB, Mechanism of Action and Metabolism

Bactericidal same mechanism of activity as rifampin (inhibits RNA polymerase). 100% cross-resistant with rifampin.

Preparation and Dose

150 mg tablets.
Dose: Adults: 600 mg once weekly during the continuation phase of treatment. (Not recommended in the US for the initial treatment phase.) Higher daily doses are being studied.
Children: (12 years and older), 600 mg once weekly if >45 kg. 450 mg once weekly if <45 kg.

Storage

Tablets should be kept at room temperature (15–25 °C).

Oral Absorption

Oral bioavailability is 70%. Peak concentration and area under the curve (AUC) are increased if given with a meal.

CSF Penetration

No information available.

Special Circumstances

Pregnancy/breastfeeding

Pregnancy category C. Use only if potential benefit outweighs possible risk.

Renal Disease

Insufficient data, but likely to be safe since only minimally excreted by the kidney.

Hepatic Disease

Pharmacokinetics are very similar to normal volunteers in persons with mild to severe liver impairment.

Adverse Effects

- Many drug interactions.
- Red-orange staining of body fluids
- Rash and pruritus
- Hypersensitivity reaction
- Hepatotoxicity
- Hematologic abnormalities.

Contraindications

History of hypersensitivity to any of the rifamycins (i.e. rifampin or rifabutin).

Monitoring

Liver function monitoring if appropriate (if given with other hepatotoxic medications or if there are symptoms of hepatotoxicity); monitor drug concentrations of interacting medications.

Alerting symptoms

- Fever
- Loss of appetite
- Malaise
- Nausea and vomiting
- Darkened urine
- Yellowish discoloration of the skin and eyes
- Pain or swelling of the joints.

LINEZOLID

Drug Class

Synthetic antimicrobial agent of the oxazolidinone class.

Mechanism of Action, Distribution, Excretion

It inhibits protein synthesis by binding to the P site of the 50S ribosomal subunit and preventing formation of the larger ribosomal — fMet-tRNA complex that initiates protein synthesis. It is 30% protein bound and distributed widely. Approximately 80% of the dose of linezolid appears in the urine.

Preparation and Dose

Linezolid is supplied as 400 mg and 600 mg tablets. The dosage for daily therapy is 600 mg once daily. Reduce to 400–300 mg/day if serious adverse effects develop. All patients should receive Vitamin B6 while receiving linezolid.

Storage

Store tablet at room temperature (15–25 °C). Reconstituted oral suspension may be stored at room temperature for 21 days.

Oral Absorption

Nearly complete oral absorption.

CSF Penetration

CSF concentration is about 1/3 of those of serum in animal models. It has been used to treat meningitis in humans.

Special Circumstances

Pregnancy/breastfeeding

It is not recommended for routine use in patients with pregnancy. It should be used during pregnancy only when benefit outweighs risk. It should be used with caution in nursing mothers.

Renal Disease

No modification in dosage in patients with renal insufficiency.

Hepatic Disease

No modification in dosage required in patients with mild to moderate hepatic disease.

Adverse Effects

Frequent

- Gastrointestinal upset
- Rash.

Rare

- Myelosuppression
- Peripheral neuropathy
- Optic neuropathy.

Contraindication

- Hypersensitivity to oxazolidinones
- Symptoms of neuropathy

Monitoring

Monitor for peripheral neuropathy, optic neuritis, complete blood count initially weekly and then monthly.

Alerting Symptoms

- Pain, numbness, tingling or weakness in extremities
- Black, tarry stools or severe diarrhea
- Unusual bleeding or bruising
- Unusual tiredness or weakness
- Headache, nausea or vomiting.

CLARITHROMYCIN

Drug Class

It is a macrolide antibiotic. Clarithromycin is a semi-synthetic derivative of erythromycin and is bacteriostatic in nature. It is usually active against nontubercular mycobacterium particularly MAC.

Mechanism of Action, Distribution and Excretion

It inhibits protein synthesis by binding reversibly to 50 S ribosomal subunits.

Distribution

It is widely distributed and achieves high intracellular concentrations. It is metabolized in liver and excreted via urine.

Preparation and Dose

Oral tablets of 250 and 500 mg. Also available in extended release tablets for once daily use.
Dose: 500 mg twice daily or 1 g daily of extended release formulation.

Adverse Effects

Frequent

- Abdominal pain
- Nausea
- Vomiting
- Occasionally diarrhea.

Rare

- Allergic skin reactions
- Liver toxicity
- QT prolongation
- *Clostridium difficile* colitis
- Hearing loss.

Special Circumstances

Pregnancy/breastfeeding

It is not recommended for routine use in patients with pregnancy. It should be used during pregnancy only when benefit outweighs risk. It should be used with caution in nursing mothers.

Renal and Hepatic Disease

Although, the pharmacokinetics of clarithromycin are altered in patients with either hepatic or renal dysfunction, dose adjustment is not necessary until the creatinine clearance is <30 mL/min.

Monitoring

No specific laboratory monitoring requirements.

Alerting Symptoms

- Severe diarrhea
- Rash.

IMIPENEM/CILASTATIN

Drug Class

Imipenem belongs to the carbapenem group of drugs. Carbapenems are betalactam antibiotics that have a broader spectrum of activity. Imipenem is derived from *Streptomyces cattleya.*

Mechanism of Action

Betalactam antibiotics interfere with the synthesis of bacterial cell wall. The beta lactam antibiotics inhibit the transpeptidases, so that cross linking of the adjacent peptide chains does not take place.

Imipenem is very resistant to hydrolysis by most beta lactamases. Activity of imipenem is excellent in vitro for a wide variety of aerobic and anaerobic microorganisms.

Pharmacokinetics

Imipenem is not absorbed orally. Imipenem is rapidly hydrolyzed by the enzyme dehydropeptidase I located on the brush border of renal tubular cells. Hence, imipenem is combined with cilastatin which is a reversible inhibitor of dehydropeptidase and thus imipenem is protected from hydrolysis.

Preparation and Dose

Lypholized powder 1:1 ratio of imipenem and cilastatin. Vials available as 250 mg, 500 mg, 750 mg, or 1 g and contain equal amounts of both drugs (i.e. a "500 mg vial" contains 500 mg of imipenem and 500 mg cilastatin).
Dose: 1,000 mg IV every 12 hours.

Storage

Powder should be kept at room temperature (15–25 °C); suspended product should be kept no more than 4 hours at room temperature or no more than 24 hours refrigerated.

CSF Penetration

Good CSF penetration, but children with meningitis treated with imipenem had high rates of seizures.

Special Circumstances

Pregnancy/breastfeeding

It should be used with caution in patients with pregnancy and breastfeeding.

Renal Disease

Dosage should be modified for patients with renal insufficiency. 750 mg every 12 hours for creatinine clearance 20–40 mL/min, 500 mg every 12 hours for creatinine clearance <20 mL/min. Dose after dialysis.

Hepatic Disease

No modification in dosage required in patients with hepatic disease.

Adverse Events

Frequent

- Diarrhea
- Nausea
- Vomiting
- Occasional.

Occasional

- Hypotension
- Thrombophlebitis
- Anemia
- Seizure (noted with CNS infection)
- Palpitations
- Pseudomembranous colitis

Contraindications

Carbapenem intolerance; meningitis (use meropenem).

Monitoring

No specific laboratory monitoring requirements.

MEROPENEM

Drug Class

Beta-lactam—carbapenem

Activity against TB, Mechanism of Action and Metabolism

In vitro activity—very limited clinical experience.

Preparation and Dose

Crystalline powder. Product is available in 500 mg, or 1 g vials.
Adults: No oral absorption. Recent case-controlled study used 1,000 mg IV every 8 hours.

Storage

Powder should be kept at room temperature (15–25 °C); suspended product should be kept no more than 4 hours at room temperature or no more than 24 hours refrigerated.

Oral Absorption

No oral absorption

CSF Penetration

Adequate CSF penetration.

Special Circumstances

Pregnancy/breastfeeding

There is little information regarding use during pregnancy; unknown safety during breastfeeding.

Renal Disease

Dose adjustment required.

Hepatic Disease

Liver disease does not alter the pharmacodynamics of meropenem.

Adverse Effects

Frequent

- Diarrhea
- Nausea or vomiting.
- Seizure (noted with CNS infection), but rare compared to imipenem.

Rare

- Elevated LFTs hematologic
- Toxicity
- Hypersensitivity.

Contraindications

Carbapenem intolerance.

Monitoring

Symptomatic monitoring.

Alerting Symptoms

- Severe diarrhea (watery or bloody)
- Skin rash, hives or itching
- Swelling in the face, throat or lips
- Wheezing or trouble breathing.

AMOXICILLIN CLAVULANATE

Drug Class

Extended spectrum semi-synthetic penicillin which is penicillinase susceptible. It is an aminopenicillin.

Mechanism of Action

Beta lactam antibiotics interfere with the synthesis of bacterial cell wall. The beta lactam antibiotics inhibit the transpeptidases, so that cross linking of the adjacent peptide chains does not take place.

Pharmacokinetics

It is not degraded by gastric acid. Primary channel of excretion is kidney. Clavulanate cleared by the liver.

Storage

Tablets are stable at room temperature (15–25 °C); reconstituted suspension should be stored in the refrigerator and discarded after 7 days.

Oral Absorption

Good oral absorption, best tolerated and well absorbed when taken at the start of a standard meal.

CSF Penetration

Approximately 5% of the plasma concentration reaches the CSF.

Special Circumstances

Pregnancy/breastfeeding

Probably safe in pregnancy (no known risk); can be used while breastfeeding.

Renal Disease

Amoxicillin is renally excreted and the dose should be adjusted for renal failure. For creatinine clearance 10–30 mL/min dose 1,000 mg as amoxicillin twice daily; for creatinine clearance <10 mL/min dose 1,000 mg as amoxicillin once daily. It is cleared by dialysis, so should be dosed after dialysis—single dose every 24 hours and after each dialysis session.

Hepatic Disease

Clavulanate is cleared by the liver, so care should be used when using in patients with liver failure.

Adverse Effects

Common

- Diarrhea
- Abdominal discomfort
- Nausea and vomiting.

Uncommon

- Hypersensitivity
- Rash
- Rare side-effects have been reported in other organ systems.

Contraindications

Penicillin allergy; use with caution with cephalosporin allergies.

Alerting Symptoms

- Rash or swelling
- Trouble breathing
- Severe diarrhea.

BEDAQUILINE

Drug Class

Diarylquinoline

Activity against TB, Mechanism of Action and Metabolism

Bactericidal, Inhibits ATP synthesis; novel method of action; the drug has a 5.5-month half-life. CYP3A4 is the major CYP isoenzyme involved in the metabolism of bedaquiline. Bedaquiline is mainly eliminated in feces. The renal clearance of unchanged drug is insignificant.

Distribution

The plasma protein binding of bedaquiline is greater than 99.9% with a high volume of distribution. The volume of distribution in the central compartment is estimated to be approximately 164 L.

Preparation and Dose

100 mg tablets.
Adults: 400 mg once daily for 2 weeks, followed by 200 mg, 3 times per week for 22 weeks with food.
Children: Not yet determined.

Storage

Store tablet at room temperature (15–25 °C).

Oral Absorption

Better absorption is obtained if taken with food.

CSF Penetration

No data are available regarding CNS penetration.

Special Circumstances

Pregnancy/breastfeeding

Not recommended during pregnancy or breastfeeding due to limited data. Reproduction studies performed in rats and rabbits have revealed no evidence of harm to the fetus.

Renal Disease

No dosage adjustment is required in patients with mild to moderate renal impairment. Dosing not established in severe renal impairment, use with caution.

Hepatic Disease

No dosage adjustment is required in patients with mild to moderate hepatic impairment. Dosing and toxicity not well established in severe hepatic impairment, use with caution and only when the benefits outweigh the risks.

Adverse Effects

Frequent

- Gastrointestinal distress (nausea, vomiting, abdominal pain, loss of appetite)
- Joint pain (arthralgia)
- Headache.

Occasional

- QT prolongation, hyperuricemia
- Phospholipidosis (the accumulation of phospholipids in the body's tissues)
- Elevated aminotransferases
- Possibly an increased risk of pancreatitis.

Contraindications

- Clinically significant ventricular arrhythmia
- A QTcF interval of >500 ms (confirmed by repeat ECG)
- Severe liver disease
- Abnormal electrolytes.

Monitoring

An ECG should be obtained before initiation of treatment, and at least 2, 4, 8, 12 and 24 weeks after starting treatment. More frequently if heart conditions, hypothyroidism or electrolyte disturbances are present. Liver function tests should be done monthly.

Alerting Symptoms

- Abdominal pain
- Yellowing of your skin or eyes
- Palpitations
- Chest pain
- Fainting and near fainting events.

DELAMANID

Drug Class

Nitrodihydro-Imidazo-Oxazole.

Activity against TB, Mechanism of Action and Metabolism

Inhibition of the synthesis of the mycobacterial cell wall components, methoxy-mycolic and keto-mycolic acid. Delamanid is a prodrug that must be reduced by the deazaflavin-dependent nitroreductase to its des-nitro metabolite to be active. The complete metabolic profile of delamanid in man has not yet been fully elucidated. Delamanid disappears from plasma with a t1/2 of 30—38 hours. Delamanid is not excreted in urine.

Distribution

It is more than 99% protein bound, with a high volume of distribution.

Preparation and Dose

50 mg film-coated tablets.
Adults: 100 mg twice daily for 24 weeks. It is recommended to administer with water and to be taken with, or just after a meal.
Children: Not yet determined.

Storage

Store tablet at room temperature and in original package.

Oral Absorption

Absorption is increased with a standard meal.

CSF Penetration

No data are available regarding CNS penetration.

Special Circumstances

Pregnancy/breastfeeding

There are very limited data from the use of delamanid in pregnant women. Studies in animals have shown reproductive toxicity. Available pharmacokinetic data in animals have shown excretion of delamanid and/or its metabolites in milk.

Renal Disease

No dosage adjustment is required in patients with mild to moderate renal impairment (dosing not established in severe renal impairment, use with caution and only when the benefits outweigh the risks).

Hepatic Disease

No dosage adjustment is required in patients with mild to moderate hepatic impairment. Dosing and toxicity not well established in severe hepatic impairment, use with caution and only when the benefits outweigh the risks

Adverse Effects

Frequent

Nausea, vomiting and dizziness.

Occasional

QT prolongation.

Contraindications

- Clinically significant ventricular arrhythmia
- A QTcF interval of >500 ms (confirmed by repeat ECG)
- Severe liver disease
- Serum albumin less than 2.8
- Abnormal electrolytes.

Monitoring

An ECG should be obtained before initiation of treatment, and at least 2, 4, 8, 12 and 24 weeks after starting treatment. Monitoring ECGs should be done monthly if taking other QT prolonging drugs (i.e. moxifloxacin, clofazimine, etc.).

Alerting Symptoms

- Palpitations
- Chest pain
- Fainting and near fainting events.

FURTHER READINGS

1. Casal M, Gutierrez J, Gonzalez J, et al. In vitro susceptibility of mycobacterium tuberculosis to a new macrolide. Am J Respir Crit Care Med. 1995;151:1083-6.
2. Chopra I, Brennam P. Molecular action of antimycobacterial agents. Tubercle Lung Dis. 1998;78:89-98.
3. Companion Handbook to the WHO guidelines for the programmatic management of drug resistant tuberculosis. WHO/HTM/TB/2014.11.
4. Davidson PJ, Le HQ. Drug treatment of tuberculosis-1992. Drugs. 1992;43:651-73.
5. De Lorenzo S, et al. Efficacy and safety of meropenem/clavulanate added to linezolid containing regimens in the treatment of MDR-/XDR-TB. European Respiratory Journal. 2013;41:1386-92.
6. Guidelines for programmatic management of drug resistant tuberculosis. WHO, 2011. WHO/HTM/TB/2011.6
7. Guidelines for the programmatic management of drug-resistant tuberculosis: emergency update 2008. Geneva, World Health Organization, 2008 (WHO/HTM/TB/ 2008.402)
8. Jagannath C, Venkta Reddy M, et al. Chemotheraputic activity of Clofazimine and its analoge against M. tuberculosis in vitro and in vivo. Am J Respir Crit Care Med. 1995;151:1083-6.
9. Lehman J. Paraaminosalicylic acid in treatment of tuberculosis. Lancet. 1946;1:15-6.

10. Sotgiu G, et al. Efficacy, safety and tolerability of linezolid containing regimens in treating MDR-TB and XDR-TB: systematic review and meta-analysis. European Respiratory Journal. 2012; 40:1430-42.
11. Sutton WB, Gordee RS, et al. In vitro and In vivo laboratory study on the antitubercular activity of capreomycin. Ann N Y Sci. 1966;135:947-59.
12. The use of bedaquiline in the treatment of multidrug-resistant tuberculosis: Interim policy guidance. Geneva:World Health Organization; 2013 (WHO/HTM/TB2013.06).
13. The use of delamanid in the treatment of multidrug-resistant tuberculosis: Interim policy guidance. Geneva:World Health Organization; 2014 (WHO/HTM/TB2014.23).

CHAPTER 5

Adverse Drug Reactions of Antitubercular Drugs Used in New Patients of TB with their Management

Adverse effects of antitubercular drugs used in new patients of tuberculosis is tabulated in Table 5.1. Symptoms based approach to management of minor and major adverse effects are tabulated in Tables 5.2 and 5.3.

TABLE 5.1: Adverse effects of antitubercular drugs used in new patients.

Sl. No.	Drug	Common adverse effect	Rare adverse effect
1.	Isoniazid	• Peripheral neuritis • Hepatotoxicity • Skin rash	• Anemia • Arthralgia • Dysarthria • Irritability • Seizure • Dysphoria • Lupoid reaction • Pellagra • Vasculitis • Thrombocytopenia • Optic neuritis
2.	Rifampicin	• Gastrointestinal reactions • Hepatitis • Orange staining of body fluids	• Flue-like syndrome • Thrombocytopenia • Hemolytic anemia • Acute renal failure • Pseudomembranous colitis • Pseudoadrenal crisis
3.	Ethambutol	• Retrobulbar neuritis	• Skin reactions • Arthralgia • Peripheral neuritis • Thrombocytopenia
4.	Pyrazinamide	• Arthralgia • Hepatotoxicity	• Gastrointestinal reaction • Cutaneous reaction • Sideroblastic anemia • Thrombocytopenia • Photosensitivity

(Contd.)

(Contd.)

Sl. No.	Drug	Common adverse effect	Rare adverse effect
5.	Streptomycin	• Vestibular and auditory nerve damage • Nephrotoxicity • Cutaneous reaction • Pain, induration at site of injection	• Hypersensitivity reaction • Anaphylactic shock • Hemolytic anemia • Aplastic anemia • Agranulocytosis • Thrombocytopenia • Electrolyte abnormalities including hypokalemia, hypocalcemia, hypomagnesemia

TABLE 5.2: Symptoms based approach to the management of minor adverse reaction not requiring stoppage of treatment.

Symptoms	Drug	Management
Abdominal pain, nausea	• Related to rifampicin	• Reassure the patients
Burning of the feet	• Related to isoniazid • Peripheral neuropathy	• Continue isoniazid, and give pyridoxine 50–75 mg daily • Large dose of pyridoxine, may interfere the action of isoniazid
Drowsiness	• Related to isoniazid	• Reassure the patients
Gastrointestinal upset	• Any oral medications	• Reassure patients • Give drugs with less water • Give drugs over longer period of time (e.g. 20 minutes) • Give drugs with small amount of food • If these measure fails, provide antiemetic
Joint pains	• Related to pyrazinamide	• Continue pyrazinamide • Use aspirin or nonsteroidal anti-inflammatory drugs • Use intermittent directly observed treatment if possible
Red urine	• Related to rifampicin	• Reassure the patients
Women on rifampicin	• Rifampicin may reduce the effectiveness of oral contraceptive pills	• Alternative method of contraception should be provided

TABLE 5.3: Symptoms based approach to major adverse effects requiring stoppage of treatment.

Symptoms	Drug	Management
Loss of hearing	• Related to streptomycin	• Otoscopy to rule out wax • Stop streptomycin if no other explanation

(Contd.)

(Contd.)

Symptoms	Drug	Management
Dizziness	• If true vertigo and nystagmus, related to streptomycin	• Stop streptomycin • If just dizziness with no nystagmus, try dose reduction for one week; If there is no improvement stop streptomycin
Generalized reactions including shock and purpura	• May be due to rifampicin, pyrazinamide and/or streptomycin, thioacetazone	• Stop all medications • Use different combination of drugs
Jaundice	• May be due to drug induced hepatitis	• Stop all antituberculosis drugs until jaundice resolves and liver enzyme revert to base levels • Reintroduce same regimen either, gradually or all at once • If hepatitis has been life-threatening and was not of viral origin it is safer to use regimen like streptomycin, ethambutol and isoniazid, fluroquinolones
Moderate to severe skin rash	• Related to all antituberculosis drugs	• Stop all antituberculosis drugs • Reintroduce drug one by one once the rash has subsided
Visual impairment	• Related to ethambutol	• Visual examination. Stop ethambutol.
Vomiting/ confusion	• Suspect drug induced hepatitis	• Urgent liver enzyme test. If liver enzyme test unavailable, stop antituberculosis drugs and observe

FURTHER READINGS

1. Byrd RB, Horn BR, Solomon DA, Griggs GA. Toxic effects of isoniazid in tuberculosis chemoprophylaxis. Role of biochemical monitoring in 1000 patients. JAMA. 1979; 241;1239-41.
2. Jhonston RN, et al. Prolonged streptomycin and isoniazid for pulmonary tuberculosis. BMJ. 1964;1:1679-83.
3. Kant S, Verma SK, Gupta V, Anand SC, Prasad R. Pyrazinamide induced thrombocytopenia. Indian J Pharmacol. 2010;42:108-9.
4. Nahid P, et al. ATS/CDC/IDSA Clinical Practice Guidelines: Treatment of Drug-Susceptible Tuberculosis. Clin Infec Dis. 2016:1-50.
5. Peloquin CA, et al. Pharmacokinetics of isoniazid under fasting condition, with food and antacids. Int J Tub and Lung Dis. 1999;3:703-10.
6. Prasad R, Mukherji PK. Ethambutol induced thrombocytopenia. Tubercle. 1989;70:211-2.
7. Prasad R, Mukherji PK. Rifampicin induced thrombocytopenia. Ind J Tub. 1989;36:44-5.
8. Steele MA, Burk RF, DesPrez RM. Toxic hepatitis with isoniazid and rifampicin: a meta-analysis. Chest. 1991;99:465-71.
9. World Health Organization. Treatment of TB Guidelines - 4th edition. WHO/HTM/TB/2009.420.

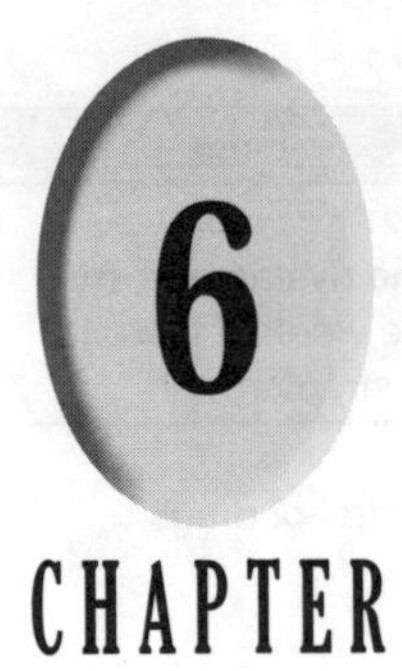

CHAPTER 6 Adverse Drug Reactions of Antitubercular Drugs Used in Drug Resistant Patients of TB with their Management

Adverse effect of antitubercular drugs used in previously treated patients of tuberculosis (TB) is tabulated in Table 6.1 and management strategy of common adverse effects are tabulated in Table 6.2.

TABLE 6.1: Adverse effects of antitubercular drugs used in previously treated TB patients.

Drug	Frequent	Occasional	Rare
Amikacin	• Pain at injection site • Proteinuria • Electrolyte disturbances (hypokalemia and hypomagnesemia)	• Cochlear ototoxicity • Vestibular toxicity • Nephrotoxicity • Peripheral neuropathy • Rash • Eosinophilia	Fever
Capreomycin	• Nephrotoxicity • Tubular dysfunction • Urticaria • Maculopapular rash	• Cochlear ototoxicity • Vestibular toxicity • Electrolyte disturbances (hypokalemia, hypomagnesemia and hypocalcemia) • Pain at injection site, induration and sterile abscesses at site of injection • Neurotoxicity	Rash
Clofazimine	• Ichthyosis • Dry skin • Pink to brown black discoloration of skin, cornea, retina and urine • Anorexia • Abdominal pain	• Hepatitis • Hypersensitivity • Nephrotoxicity • Acneiform eruption	Phototoxicity

(Contd.)

(Contd.)

Drug	Frequent	Occasional	Rare
Cycloserine and teridazone	• Neurological disturbances (headache and tremors) • Psychiatric disturbances (sleep disturbances, anxiety, depression, irritability, confusion, drowsiness) • Inflammation of gums • Pale skin	• Visual changes and eye pain • Skin rash • Jaundice (hepatitis) • Burning, tingling and numbness in hands and feet	• Seizures • Suicidal thoughts • Impaired hearing in fetus • Hypersensitivity
Ethionamide and prothionamide	• Severe gastrointestinal intolerance (including nausea, vomiting, diarrhea, abdominal pain, excessive salivation metallic taste) • Dose related headache • Anorexia and weight loss • Stomatitis	• Neurological disturbances • Psychiatric disturbances (depression, restlessness, drowsiness) • Allergic reactions • Postural hypotension • Reversible hepatitis (transient increase in serum bilirubin) • Hypothyroidism (especially when combined with PAS) • Menstrual irregularity • Gynecomastia • Arthralgias • Leukopenia	• Peripheral neuritis • Optic neuritis • Pellagra-like syndrome • Rash • Photosensitivity • Thrombocyt-openia • Alopecia • Impotence • Purpura
Kanamycin	• Pain at injection site • Renal damage (usually reversible)	• Cochlear and vestibular ototoxicity (usually irreversible) • Peripheral neuropathy • Rash • Nephrotoxicity (dose related to cumulative and peak concentration, often irreversible)	Fever

(Contd.)

(Contd.)

Drug	Frequent	Occasional	Rare
Gatifloxacin	Generally well tolerated	• Gastrointestinal intolerance	• Headache • Malaise • Insomnia • Restlessness • Dizziness • Diarrhea • Photosensitivity • Tendon rupture • Dysglycemia • Increase liver function test
Levofloxacin	• Generally well tolerated	• Gastrointestinal intolerance (diarrhea) • Neurological disturbances (insomnia, restlessness, dizziness) • Allergic reactions • Photosensitivity	• QT prolongation • Peripheral neuropathy • Tendon rupture • Rash
Moxifloxacin	• Generally well tolerated	• Gastrointestinal intolerance (diarrhea) • Neurological disturbances (insomnia, restlessness, dizziness) • Allergic reactions • Photosensitivity	• QT prolongation (in isolated cases) • Rash
Ofloxacin	• Generally well tolerated	• Gastrointestinal intolerance (diarrhea) • Neurological disturbances (headache, insomnia, restlessness)	• Allergic reactions • Photosensitivity • Peripheral neuropathy • Tendon rupture • Increased liver function tests
Para-amino-salicylic acid (PAS)	• Gastrointestinal intolerance (including metallic taste, anorexia, diarrhea) • Hypothyroidism especially when combined with ethionamide	• Hepatitis • Thyroid enlargement • Allergic reactions • Fever • Increased prothrombin time • Malabsorption syndrome (e.g. steatorrhea and low serum folate level)	

(Contd.)

(Contd.)

Drug	Frequent	Occasional	Rare
Linezolid	• Gastrointestinal intolerance • Rash • Headache	• Myelosuppression • Peripheral neuropathy • Optic neuropathy	
Clarithromycin	• Gastrointestinal intolerance (abdominal pain, nausea, vomiting, diarrhea) • Hepatitis • Ventricular arrhythmias		• Hypersensitivity reaction • Pseudomembranous colitis • Fever • Rash
Refabutin	• Hepatitis • Leukopenia • Rashes	Skin discoloration (Bronzing or pseudo-jaundice)	• Thrombocytopenia • Anterior uveitis
Imipenem/ cilastatin	• Gastrointestinal intolerance • Hypersensitivity reaction • Palpitation • Tachycardia	• Seizure • Hypotension • Anemia • Thrombophlebitis	• Renal failure • Hemorrhagic colitis • Pseudomembranous colitis
Meropenem	• Diarrhea • Nausea • Vomiting	• Seizure (in CNS infection)	• Elevated LFT • Hematologic toxicity
Thiacetazone	• Gastrointestinal intolerance • Rash • Anemia	• Hepatitis • Exfoliative dermatitis • Stevens-Johnson syndrome	• Bone marrow depression • Ototoxicity
Amoxicillin/ clavulanate	• Diarrhea • Rash • Hypersensitivity reaction	• Candida stomatitis • Vaginitis	• Hepatic injury
Bedaquiline	• Gastrointestinal distress (nausea, vomiting, abdominal pain, loss of appetite) • Joint pain • Headache	• QT prolongation • Hyperuricemia	
Delamanid	• Nausea • Vomiting • Dizziness	• QT prolongation	

TABLE 6.2: Common adverse effects, suspected agent(s) and management strategies of antituberculous drugs used in drug resistant TB.

Adverse effect	Suspected agent	Suggested management strategies
Seizures	**CS** H Fq	• Suspend suspected agent pending resolution of seizures • Initiate anticonvulsant therapy (e.g. phenytoin, valproic acid) • Increase pyridoxine to maximum daily dose (200 mg per day) • Restart suspected agent or reinitiate suspected agent at lower dose, if essential to the regimen • Discontinue suspected agent if this can be done without compromising regimen • Anticonvulsant is generally continued until MDR-TB treatment is completed or suspected agent discontinued • History of previous seizure disorder is not a contraindication to the use of agents listed here if a patient's seizures are well controlled and/or the patient is receiving anticonvulsant • Patients with history of previous seizures may be at increased risk for development of seizures during MDR-TB treatment
Peripheral neuropathy	**CS** **Lzd** **H** S Km Am Cm Eto/Pto Fq	• Increase pyridoxine to maximum daily dose (200 mg per day) • Change injectable to capreomycin if patient has documented susceptibility to capreomycin • Initiate therapy with tricyclic antidepressants such as amitriptyline. Nonsteroidal anti-inflammatory drugs or acetaminophen may help alleviate symptoms • Lower dose of suspected agent, if this can be done without compromising regimen • Discontinue suspected agent if this can be done without compromising regimen • Patients with comorbid disease (e.g. diabetes, HIV, alcohol neuropathy (dependence) may be more likely to develop peripheral neuropathy, but these conditions are not contraindications to the use of the agents • Neuropathy may be irreversible; however, some patients may experience improvement when offending agents are suspended

(Contd.)

(Contd.)

Adverse effect	Suspected agent	Suggested management strategies
Hearing loss	**S** **Km** **Am** **Cm** Clr	• Document hearing loss and compare with baseline audiometry if available • Change parenteral treatment to capreomycin if patient has documented susceptibility to capreomycin • Decrease frequency and/or lower dose of suspected agent if this can be done without compromising the regimen (consider administration three times per week) • Discontinue suspected agent if this can be done without compromising the regimen • Patients with previous exposure to aminoglycosides may have baseline hearing loss. In such patients, audiometry may be helpful at the start of MDR-TB therapy • Hearing loss is generally not reversible • The risk of further hearing loss must be weighed against the risks of stopping the injectable in the treatment regimen • While the benefit of hearing aids is minimal to moderate in auditory toxicity, consider a trial use to determine if a patient with hearing loss can benefit from their use
Psychotic symptoms	**Cs** **H** Fq Eto/Pto	• Stop suspected agent for a short period of time (1–4 weeks) while psychotic symptoms are brought under control • Initiate antipsychotic therapy • Lower dose of suspected agent if this can be done without compromising regimen • Discontinue suspected agent if this can be done without compromising regimen • Some patients will need to continue antipsychotic treatment throughout MDR-TB therapy • Previous history of psychiatric disease is not a contraindication to the use of agents listed here but may increase the likelihood of psychotic symptoms developing during treatment • Psychotic symptoms are generally reversible upon completion of MDR-TB treatment or cessation of the offending agent
Depression	**Cs** Fq Eto/Pto H	• Offer group or individual counseling • Initiate antidepressant therapy • Lower dose of suspected agent if this can be done without compromising regimen • Discontinue suspected agent if this can be done without compromising regimen • Socioeconomic conditions and chronic illness should not be underestimated as contributing factors to depression

(Contd.)

(Contd.)

Adverse effect	Suspected agent	Suggested management strategies
		• Depressive symptoms may fluctuate during therapy and may improve as illness is successfully treated • History of previous depression is not a contraindication to the use of the agents listed but may increase the likelihood of depression developing during treatment
Hypothyroidism	**PAS** **Eto/Pto**	• Initiate thyroxine therapy • Completely reversible upon discontinuation of PAS or ethionamide/prothionamide • The combination of ethionamide/ prothionamide with PAS is more frequently associated with hypothyroidism than the individual use of each drug
Nausea and vomiting	**Eto/Pto** **PAS** H E Z Bdq Dlm	• Assess for dehydration; initiate rehydration if indicated • Initiate antiemetic therapy • Lower dose of suspected agent if this can be done without compromising regimen • Discontinue suspected agent if this can be done without compromising regimen rarely necessary • Nausea and vomiting universal in early weeks of therapy and usually abate with time on treatment and adjunctive therapy • Electrolytes should be monitored if vomiting is severe • Reversible upon discontinuation of suspected agent • Severe abdominal distress and acute abdomen have been reported with the use of clofazimine. Although these reports are rare, if this effect occurs, clofazimine should be suspended
Gastritis	**PAS** **Eto/Pto** Bdq Dlm	• H2-blockers, proton-pump inhibitors, or antacids • Stop suspected agent(s) for short periods of time (e.g. 1–7 days) • Lower dose of suspected agent, if this can be done without compromising regimen • Discontinue suspected agent if this can be done without compromising regimen • Severe gastritis, as manifested by hematemesis, melena or hematochezia, is rare • Dosing of antacids should be carefully timed so as to not interfere with the absorption of antituberculosis drugs (take 2 hours before or 3 hours after antituberculosis medications) • Reversible upon discontinuation of suspected agent(s)

(Contd.)

(Contd.)

Adverse effect	Suspected agent	Suggested management strategies
Hepatitis	**Z** **H** **R** Eto/Pto PAS Fq	• Stop all therapy pending resolution of hepatitis • Eliminate other potential causes of hepatitis • Consider suspending most likely agent permanently • Reintroduce remaining drugs, one at a time while monitoring liver function • History of previous hepatitis should be carefully analyzed to determine most likely causative agent(s); these should be avoided in future regimens • Generally reversible upon discontinuation of suspected agent
Renal toxicity	**S** **Km** **Am** **Cm**	• Discontinue suspected agent • Consider using capreomycin if an aminoglycoside had been the prior injectable in regimen • Consider dosing 2–3 times a week if drug is essential to the regimen and patient can tolerate (close monitoring of creatinine) • Adjust all antituberculosis medications according to the creatinine clearance • History of diabetes or renal disease is not a contraindication to the use of the agents listed here, although patients with these comorbidities may be at increased risk for developing renal failure • Renal impairment may be permanent
Electrolyte disturbances (hypokalemia and hypomagnesemia)	**Cm** **Km** **Am** S	• Check potassium • If potassium is low, also check magnesium (and calcium if hypocalcemia is suspected) • Replace electrolytes as needed • If severe hypokalemia is present, consider hospitalization • Amiloride 5–10 mg QD or spironolactone 25 mg QD may decrease potassium and magnesium wasting and is useful in refractory cases • Oral potassium replacements can cause significant nausea and vomiting. Oral magnesium may cause diarrhea
Optic neuritis	**E** Eto/Pto	• Stop E • Refer patient to an ophthalmologist • Usually reverses with cessation of E • Rare case reports of optic neuritis have been attributed to streptomycin

(Contd.)

(Contd.)

Adverse effect	Suspected agent	Suggested management strategies
Arthralgias	**Z** Fq Bdq	• Initiate therapy with nonsteroidal anti-inflammatory drugs • Lower dose of suspected agent if this can be done without compromising regimen • Discontinue suspected agent if this can be done without compromising regimen • Symptoms of arthralgia generally diminish over time, even without intervention • Uric acid levels may be elevated in patients on pyrazinamide. Allopurinol appears not to correct the uric acid levels in such cases

(H: isoniazid; R: rifampicin; E: ethambutol; Z: pyrazinamide; S: streptomycin; Km: kanamycin; Am: amikacin; Cm: capreomycin; Fq: fluoroquinolones; Eto: ethionamide; Pto: prothionamide; PAS: para-aminosalicylic acid; Cs: cycloserine; Cfz: clofazimine; Lzd: linezolid; Clr: clarithromycin; Bdq: bedaquiline; Dlm: delamanid; MDR-TB: multidrug resistant tuberculosis).

Note: Drugs that the strongly associated with adverse effects shown in bold.

FURTHER READINGS

1. Casal M, Gutierrez J, Gonzalez J, et al. In vitro susceptibility of mycobacterium tuberculosis to a new macrolide. Am J Respir Crit Care Med. 1995;151:1083-6.
2. Chopra I, Brennam P. Molecular action of antimycobacterial agents. Tubercle Lung Dis. 1998;78:89-98.
3. Companion Handbook to the WHO guidelines for the programmatic management of drug resistant tuberculosis. WHO/HTM/TB/2014.11.
4. Davidson PJ, Le HQ. Drug treatment of tuberculosis-1992. Drugs. 1992;43:651-73.
5. De Lorenzo S, et al. Efficacy and safety of meropenem/clavulanate added to linezolid containing regimens in the treatment of MDR-/XDR-TB. E R J. 2013; 41:1386-92.
6. Guidelines for programmatic management of drug resistant tuberculosis. WHO, 2011. WHO/HTM/TB/2011.6
7. Guidelines for the programmatic management of drug-resistant tuberculosis: emergency update 2008. Geneva, World Health Organization, 2008 (WHO/HTM/TB/ 2008.402)
8. Jagannath C, Venkta Reddy M, et al. Chemotheraputic activity of Clofazimine and its analoge against M.tuberculosis in vitro and in vivo. Am J Respir Crit Care Med. 1995;151:1083-6.
9. Lehman J. Paraaminosalicylic acid in treatment of tuberculosis. Lancet. 1946;1:15-6.
10. Nahid P, et al. ATS/CDC/IDSA Clinical Practice Guidelines: Treatment of Drug-Susceptible Tuberculosis. Clin Infec Dis. 2016:1-50.
11. Sutton WB, Gordee RS, et al. In vitro and In vivo laboratory study on the antitubercular activity of capreomycin. Ann N Y Sci. 1966;135:947-59.

CHAPTER 7 Drug Interactions of Antitubercular Drugs Used in New Patients of Tuberculosis

DRUG INTERACTIONS OF ISONIAZID

Foods

Isoniazid should be taken preferably on an empty stomach because it requires an acid medium in order to be absorbed. Foods, particularly carbohydrates, can decrease the absorption of the drug by as much as 57% and the plasma concentration of the drug by as much as 30%. The drug should not be taken with fluids containing excess glucose or lactose. Isoniazid inhibits the monoamine oxidase enzyme and should not be taken concomitantly with foods rich in tyramine and histamine, such as certain types of cheese (Swiss and Cheshire), fish (tuna and herring), and alcohol, especially red wine. The symptoms of these interactions include palpitation, sweating, flushing of the face, chills, headache, diarrhea, erythema, and pruritus.

Antacids

Drugs that increase the gastric pH delay the absorption of isoniazid. Antacids containing aluminum hydroxide or ranitidine should be administered one hour after the administration of isoniazid.

Other Drugs

Isoniazid is an inhibitor of the cytochrome P450 (CYP450) system families CYP2C9, CYP2C19, and CYP2E1, but its effect on the CYP3A family is minimal. This inhibitory effect of isoniazid can increase the plasma concentrations of certain drugs to toxic levels. The plasma concentrations of anticonvulsants, such as phenytoin and carbamazepine, can increase when these drugs are used in combination with isoniazid. The same occurs with the benzodiazepines that are metabolized by oxidation (e.g. diazepam), as well as with theophylline, valproic acid, disulfiram, acetaminophen, and oral anticoagulants. The combination of isoniazid and levodopa can cause hypertension, palpitation, and flushing of the face.

Para-aminosalicylic acid (PAS) competes with the acetylation of isoniazid and prolongs half-life.

DRUG INTERACTIONS OF RIFAMPICIN

Foods

Rifampicin should be taken on an empty stomach. Foods decrease the absorption of the drug by as much as 26%, as well as increasing the time required for the drug to reach maximum concentration and decreasing that concentration by 15–36%.

Antacids

Antacids containing aluminum hydroxide delay the absorption of rifampicin.

Other Drugs

A large number of interactions can occur between rifampicin and other drugs. The drug is a potent inducer of the CYP450 system, including the CYP3A and CYP2C subfamilies, which account for more than 80% of the CYP450 isoenzymes. Therefore, rifampicin can increase the metabolism of numerous drugs that are partially or completely metabolized by CYP450 when these drugs are administered concomitantly with rifampicin. In addition, rifampicin induces uridine diphosphate-glucuronosyltransferase, an enzyme that has also been implicated in the metabolism of various drugs, the plasma levels of which can be reduced when such drugs are administered in combination with rifampicin. The possibility of interaction between rifampicin and other drugs calls for a thorough history taking that focuses on the drugs currently used by patients. There is a decrease in the plasma concentrations of the following drugs when administered concomitantly with rifampicin: oral hypoglycemic agents, the doses of which might have to be increased, and which might sometimes have to be replaced with insulin; protease inhibitors and non-nucleoside reverse transcriptase inhibitors, although efavirenz or a combination of saquinavir and ritonavir can be used without the need for discontinuing rifampicin; oral anticoagulants, the doses of which should be carefully monitored, as should their international normalized ratios; and other drugs, such as valproic acid, antidepressants (nortriptyline and sertraline), barbiturates, benzodiazepines, beta-adrenergic blocking agents, ketoconazole, chloramphenicol, contraceptives, corticosteroids, cyclosporine, dapsone, digoxin, diltiazem, enalapril, phenytoin, fluconazole, haloperidol, itraconazole, macrolides, nifedipine, quinidine, rapamycin, simvastatin, theophylline, and verapamil. The administration of rifampicin in combination with ketoconazole or PAS acid decreases the serum levels of rifampicin. The drugs should be administered separately, at least 12 hours apart.

Newer derivatives of rifampicin like rifabutin and rifapentene with longer half-life has less effect on the pharmacokinetics of antiretroviral drugs. Rifampicin reduces the effectiveness of oral contraceptive so contraceptive failures have occurred and patients should be advised to switch over to an oral contraceptive containing higher dose (50 µg) of estrogen or use alternative method of contraception.

DRUG INTERACTIONS OF PYRAZINAMIDE

Foods

Foods have very little impact on the absorption of pyrazinamide. The drug can be taken at mealtime.

Antacids

Antacids do not interfere with the absorption of pyrazinamide.

Other Drugs

Probenecid, rifampicin, isoniazid, and ethionamide can potentiate the toxic effects of pyrazinamide. The combination of pyrazinamide and zidovudine can reduce the effect of pyrazinamide. Pyrazinamide antagonizes the effects of probenecid and decreases the serum concentration of cyclosporine. Pyrazinamide can increase the serum concentrations of uric acid, and it might be necessary to adjust the doses of allopurinol and colchicine in patients under gout treatment.

DRUG INTERACTIONS OF ETHAMBUTOL

Foods

Foods have a minimal effect on the bioavailability of ethambutol.

Antacids

Antacids can reduce the maximum concentration of ethambutol by as much as 28%. The drugs should therefore be administered at longer intervals.

Other Drugs

Ethionamide can exacerbate the toxic effects of ethambutol.

DRUG INTERACTIONS OF STREPTOMYCIN

Other Drugs

The ototoxicity and nephrotoxicity of streptomycin can be potentiated by concomitant administration of amphotericin B, vancomycin, cephalosporin, cisplatin, and loop diuretics (ethacrynic acid and furosemide).

Streptomycin can themselves potentiate the effects of neuromuscular blocking agents. Concomitant administration of streptomycin and neuromuscular blocking agents can cause respiratory depression due to respiratory muscle weakness. Patients with myasthenia gravis, botulism, hypocalcemia, severe hypokalemia, or hypomagnesemia are particularly susceptible to such adverse effects. The interaction between streptomycin and neuromuscular blocking agents is independent of the order of their administration. Patients using aminoglycosides should be monitored for the occurrence of respiratory depression in the perioperative and postoperative periods. In vitro inactivation of penicillin (possible). Do not mix penicillin and streptomycin before administration. Thiacetazone can potentiate the ototoxicity of streptomycin.

FURTHER READINGS

1. Baciewicz AM, Chrisman CR, Finch CK, Self TH. Update on rifampicin and rifabutin drug interactions. Am J Med Sci. 2008;335:126-36.
2. Blumberg HM, Burman WJ, Chaisson RE, Daley CL, Etkind SC, Friedman LN, et al. American Thoracic Society/Centers for Disease Control and Prevention/Infectious Diseases Society of America: treatment of tuberculosis. Am J Respir Crit Care Med. 2003;167:603-62.
3. Caminero Luna JA. Guía de la. Tuberculosis para Médicos Especialistas. Paris: Unión Internacional Contra la Tuberculosis y Enfermedades Respiratorias; 2003.
4. Chemotherapy and management of tuberculosis in the United Kingdom: recommendations 1998. Joint Tuberculosis Committee of the British Thoracic Society. Thorax. 1998;53:536-48.
5. Desta Z, Soukhova NV, Flockhart DA. Inhibition of cytochrome P450 (CYP450) isoforms by isoniazid: potent inhibition of CYP2C19 and CYP3A. Antimicrob Agents Chemother. 2001;45:382-92.
6. Dooley KE, Chaisson RE. Tuberculosis and diabetes mellitus: convergence of two epidemics. Lancet Infect Dis. 2009;9:737-46.
7. Engelhard D, Stutman HR, Marks MI. Interaction of ketoconazole with rifampicin and isoniazid. N Engl J Med. 1984;311:1681-3.
8. Migliori GB, D, Arcy Richardson M, Sotgiu G, Lange C. Multidrug-resistant and extensively drug-resistant tuberculosis in the West. Europe and United States: epidemiology, surveillance, and control. Clin Chest Med. 2009;30:637-65, vii.
9. Nahid P, et al. ATS/CDC/IDSA Clinical Practice Guidelines: Treatment of Drug-Susceptible Tuberculosis. Clin Infec Dis. 2016:1-50.
10. Niemi M, Backman JT, Fromm MF, Neuvonen PJ, Kivistö KT. Pharmacokinetic interactions with rifampicin: clinical relevance. Clin Pharmacokinet. 2003;42:819-50.
11. Pai MP, Momary KM, Rodvold KA. Antibiotic drug interactions. Med Clin North Am. 2006;90:1223-55.
12. Self TH, Chrisman CR, Baciewicz AM, Bronze MS. Isoniazid drug and food interactions. Am J Med Sci. 1999;317:304-11.
13. World Health Organization. Treatment of TB Guidelines - 4th edition. WHO/HTM/TB/2009.420
14. World Health Organization. Treatment of Tuberculosis: Guidelines for National Programmes. Geneva: World Health Organization; 2003, 2009.
15. Yew WW. Clinically significant interactions with drugs used in the treatment of tuberculosis. Drug Saf. 2002;25:111-33.

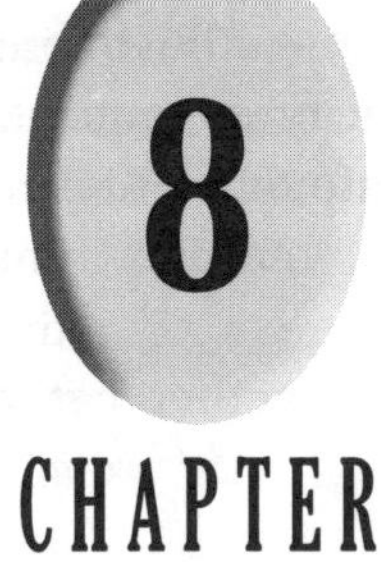

CHAPTER 8

Drug Interactions of Antitubercular Drugs Used in Drug Resistant Patients of Tuberculosis

DRUG INTERACTIONS OF KANAMYCIN

Loop diuretics (bumetanide, furosemide, ethacrynic acid, torasemide): Coadministration of aminoglycosides with loop diuretics may have an additive or synergistic auditory ototoxicity. Ototoxicity appears to be dose-dependent and may be increased with renal dysfunction. Irreversible ototoxicity has been reported. Avoid concomitant administration; if used together, careful dose adjustments in patients with renal failure and close monitoring for ototoxicity are required.

Non-depolarizing muscle relaxants (atracurium, pancuronium, tubocurarine, gallamine triethiodide): Possible enhanced action of non-depolarizing muscle relaxant resulting in possible respiratory depression. Avoid coadministration; if concurrent administration is needed, titrate the non-depolarizing muscle relaxant slowly and monitor neuromuscular function closely.

Nephrotoxic agents (amphotericin B, foscarnet, cidofovir): Additive nephrotoxicity. Avoid coadministration; if used together, monitor renal function closely and discontinue if warranted.

Penicillins: In vitro inactivation (possible). Do not mix together before administration.

DRUG INTERACTIONS OF AMIKACIN

Loop diuretics (bumetanide, furosemide, ethacrynic acid, torasemide): Coadministration of aminoglycosides with loop diuretics may have an additive or synergistic auditory ototoxicity. Ototoxicity appears to be dose-dependent and may be increased with renal dysfunction. Irreversible ototoxicity has been reported. Avoid concomitant administration; if used together, careful dose adjustments in patients with renal failure and close monitoring for ototoxicity are required.

Non-depolarizing muscle relaxants (atracurium, pancuronium, tubocurarine, gallamine triethiodide): Possible enhanced action of non-

depolarizing muscle relaxants resulting in possible respiratory depression. Avoid concomitant administration; if used together, careful dose adjustments in patients with renal failure and close monitoring for ototoxicity are required.
Nephrotoxic agents (amphotericin B, foscarnet, cidofovir): Additive nephrotoxicity. Avoid coadministration; if used together, monitor renal function closely and discontinue if warranted.
Penicillins: In vitro inactivation (possible). Do not mix together before administration.

DRUG INTERACTIONS OF CAPREOMYCIN

Avoid coadministration of non-depolarizing muscle relaxants. If concurrent administration is needed, titrate the non-depolarizing muscle relaxant slowly and monitor neuromuscular function closely. Though not reported with capreomycin, neuromuscular blockade has been reported with other polypeptide antibiotics when administered with non-depolarizing muscle relaxants. Avoid use with other nephro- or ototoxic agents because of the additive effect.

DRUG INTERACTIONS OF ETHIONAMIDE AND PROTHIONAMIDE

Foods

The effects of foods on the bioavailability of ethionamide are minimal.

Antacids

Antacids do not interfere with the absorption of ethionamide.

Other Drugs

Concomitant use of ethionamide and cycloserine/terizidone or isoniazid can potentiate the neurotoxic effects like hallucinations, irritability, tremors, depression, convulsions, psychosis, and peripheral neuropathy. Concomitant use of ethionamide and para-aminosalicylic acid (PAS) can increase hepatotoxicity and the possibility of hypothyroidism. Concomitant use of ethionamide and alcohol can produce psychotic reactions.

DRUG INTERACTIONS OF CYCLOSERINE/TERIZIDONE

Foods

Foods increase the time required for cycloserine/terizidone to be absorbed by 3.5 times, and there can be a 35% reduction in the maximum concentration of the drug. Orange juice and probably other acidic beverages reduces the maximum concentration of the drug by 15%. Whenever possible, the drug should be ingested with water, well before or after meals.

Antacids

Antacids do not significantly interfere with the absorption and concentration of cycloserine/terizidone.

Other Drugs

There is evidence that combining cycloserine/terizidone with ethionamide and isoniazid can potentiate the neurotoxic effects. Cycloserine/terizidone can increase the serum levels of phenytoin and oral anticoagulants, as well as decreasing those of pyridoxine. In patients using anticonvulsants and neuroleptics, the dose of cycloserine/terizidone should be adjusted. However, due to the potential effect that cycloserine/terizidone has on the central nervous system, patients should be closely monitored for side effects of this drug combination. Concomitant use of cycloserine/terizidone and fluoroquinolones can worsen the effects on the central nervous system (CNS). Concomitant use of cycloserine/terizidone and alcohol increases the risk of convulsions. Vitamin B6 decreases CNS effects.

DRUG INTERACTIONS OF PARA-AMINOSALICYLIC ACID (PAS)

Foods

Foods increase the absorption of PAS. The drug can be administered with water, orange juice, or fatty foods.

Antacids

Antacids do not interfere with the absorption of PAS.

Other Drugs

Digoxin can reduce the absorption of PAS and can also decrease digoxin absorption, monitor digoxin level and digoxin may need to be increased. Ethionamide can increase hepatotoxicity and hypothyroidism in patients treated with PAS. It may decrease acetylation of isoniazid resulting in increased isoniazid level. Dose of isoniazid may need to be decreased. Concomitant use of angiotensin-converting enzyme inhibitors and PAS can reduce the antihypertensive effect, and the use of calcium channel blockers can increase the anticoagulant effect of PAS. Concomitant use of PAS and carbonic anhydrase inhibitors potentiate the adverse effects of both drugs, and concomitant use of PAS and systemic corticosteroids can also increase the number and severity of adverse effects, especially gastrointestinal effects. PAS can reduce the effect of loop diuretics, and, conversely, loop diuretics can increase the serum levels of PAS. With the exception of diclofenac, nonselective nonsteroidal anti-inflammatory drugs NSAIDs can increase the adverse effects of PAS. Para-aminosalicylic acid can increase the hypoglycemic effects of sulfonylurea, as well as increasing the risk of bleeding when administered in conjunction with oral anticoagulants, thrombolytics, or salicylates.

DRUG INTERACTIONS OF LEVOFLOXACIN

Foods

Foods, with the exception of dairy products with a high concentration of calcium, do not interfere with the absorption of levofloxacin as they do with the absorption of other fluoroquinolones. Patients using ciprofloxacin should be instructed to avoid excessive use of foods with high caffeine content, since ciprofloxacin inhibits the cytochrome P450 system, thereby reducing caffeine clearance.

Antacids

Antacids containing calcium, aluminum, or magnesium interfere with the absorption and concentration of levofloxacin. Sucralfate inhibits the absorption of the drugs. Levofloxacin should not be administered until 2 hours after the use of antacids. The administration of H_2 receptor blockers does not interfere with the absorption of levofloxacin.

Other Drugs

Vitamin supplements containing zinc or iron interfere with the gastrointestinal absorption of levofloxacin. Formation of fluoroquinolone-ion complex results in decreased absorption of levofloxacin. Fluoroquinolones can inhibit numerous cytochrome P450 subfamilies, which increases the plasma concentrations of drugs that are metabolized via the cytochrome P450 system. Fluoroquinolones increase the serum levels of theophylline, glibenclamide, and cyclosporine, as well as increasing the effect of oral anticoagulants. Levofloxacin do not inhibit the cytochrome P450 enzyme system and therefore do not interact with the aforementioned drugs. However, when a levofloxacin is concomitantly administered with oral anticoagulants, the international normalized ratio should be closely monitored. Probenecid and cimetidine can increase the serum levels of levofloxacin. Concomitant administration of levofloxacin and NSAIDs can increase central nervous system stimulation and the possibility of convulsions. Levofloxacin should not be given to patients receiving class Ia antiarrhythmic drugs (such as quinidine and procainamide) or Class III antiarrhythmics (such as amiodarone and sotalol). Probenecid interferes with renal tubular secretion of fluoroquinolones, which may result in 50% increase in serum level of levofloxacin. Levofloxacin may inhibit cytochrome P450 1A2 resulting in increased mexiletine concentration.

DRUG INTERACTIONS OF MOXIFLOXACIN

Foods

Foods, with the exception of dairy products with a high concentration of calcium do not interfere with the absorption of moxifloxacin as they do with the absorption of other fluoroquinolones.

Antacids

Antacids containing calcium, aluminum, or magnesium interfere with the absorption and concentration of fluoroquinolones. Sucralfate inhibits the absorption of the drugs. Moxifloxacin should not be administered until 2 hours after the use of antacids. The administration of H_2 receptor blockers does not interfere with the absorption of moxifloxacin.

Other Drugs

Vitamin supplements containing zinc or iron interfere with the gastrointestinal absorption of moxifloxacin. Formation of fluoroquinolone-ion complex results in decreased absorption of moxifloxacin. Fluoroquinolones can inhibit numerous cytochrome P450 subfamilies, which increases the plasma concentrations of drugs that are metabolized via the cytochrome P450 system. Fluoroquinolones in general increase the serum levels of theophylline, glibenclamide, and cyclosporine, as well as increasing the effect of oral anticoagulants. Moxifloxacin do not inhibit the cytochrome P450 enzyme system and therefore do not interact with the aforementioned drugs. However, when a moxifloxacin is concomitantly administered with oral anticoagulants, the international normalized ratio should be closely monitored. Probenecid and cimetidine can increase the serum levels of moxifloxacin. Concomitant administration of moxifloxacin and NSAIDs can increase central nervous system stimulation and the possibility of convulsions. Moxifloxacin Should not be given to patients receiving class Ia antiarrhythmic drugs (such as quinidine and procainamide) or class III antiarrhythmics (such as amiodarone and sotalol).

DRUG INTERACTIONS OF OFLOXACIN

Foods

Foods, with the exception of dairy products with a high concentration of calcium do not interfere with the absorption of ofloxacin as they do with the absorption of other fluoroquinolones.

Antacids

Antacids containing calcium, aluminum, or magnesium interfere with the absorption and concentration of ofloxacin. Sucralfate inhibits the absorption of the drugs. Ofloxacin should not be administered until 2 hours after the use of antacids. The administration of H_2 receptor blockers does not interfere with the absorption of ofloxacin.

Other Drugs

Fluoroquinolones are known to inhibit hepatic drug metabolism and may interfere with the clearance of drugs such as theophylline and caffeine that are metabolized by the liver. The urinary excretion of ofloxacin and some other fluoroquinolones is reduced by probenecid; plasma concentrations are not necessarily increased. When a fluoroquinolone is concomitantly administered with oral anticoagulants, the international normalized ratio (INR) should be closely monitored. Probenecid and cimetidine can increase the serum levels of fluoroquinolones. Concomitant administration of fluoroquinolones and NSAIDs can increase CNS stimulation and the possibility of convulsions.

DRUG INTERACTIONS OF AMOXICILLIN CLAVULANIC ACID

Foods

Co-amoxiclav can be given without regard to meals. Absorption of clavulanate potassium when taken with food is greater relative to the fasted state. Co-amoxiclav should be taken at the start of a meal to enhance the absorption of amoxicillin and to minimize the potential for gastrointestinal intolerance. It is not recommended to be taken with a high fat meal, because clavulanate absorption is decreased.

Antacids

The pharmacokinetics of amoxicillin and clavulanate were not affected by administration of an antacid, either simultaneously with or 2 hours.

Other Drugs

Probenecid

Probenecid decreases the renal tubular secretion of amoxicillin but does not delay renal excretion of clavulanic acid. Concurrent use with amoxicillin clavulunate may result in increased and prolonged blood concentrations of amoxicillin. Coadministration of probenecid is not recommended.

Oral Anticoagulants

Abnormal prolongation of prothrombin time INR has been reported in patients receiving amoxicillin and oral anticoagulants. Appropriate monitoring should be undertaken when anticoagulants are prescribed concurrently with amoxicillin clavulanate. Adjustments in the dose of oral anticoagulants may be necessary to maintain the desired level of anticoagulation.

Allopurinol

The concurrent administration of allopurinol and amoxicillin increases the incidence of rashes in patients receiving both drugs as compared to patients receiving amoxicillin alone. It is not known whether this potentiation of amoxicillin rashes is due to allopurinol or the hyperuricemia present in these patients.

Oral Contraceptives

Amoxicillin clavulunate may affect intestinal flora, leading to lower estrogen reabsorption and reduced efficacy of combined oral estrogen/progesterone contraceptives.

Effects on Laboratory Tests

High urine concentrations of amoxicillin may result in false-positive reactions when testing for the presence of glucose in urine using Clinitest, Benedict's solution, or Fehling's solution. Since this effect may also occur with amoxicillin clavulanate, it is recommended that glucose tests based on enzymatic glucose oxidase reactions be used.

Pregnancy

Following administration of amoxicillin to pregnant women, a transient decrease in plasma concentration of total conjugated estriol, estriol-glucuronide, conjugated estrone, and estradiol has been noted.

DRUG INTERACTIONS OF LINEZOLID

Foods

Avoid foods or drinks with high tyramine content during use because the combination may cause a serious rise in your blood pressure. Foods high in tyramine include those that may change as a result of aging, fermentation, pickling, or smoking. The tyramine content of any protein-rich food (meat, fish and dairy products) may increase if stored for long periods or improperly refrigerated. Some foods high in tyramine include aged cheeses (0–15 milligrams per ounce); fermented or air-dried meats (0.1–8 milligrams per ounce); sauerkraut (8 milligrams per 8 ounces); soy sauce (5 milligrams per 1 teaspoon); tap beers (4 milligrams per 12 ounces); red wines (0–6 milligrams per 8 ounces). Total intake of tyramine should be less than 100 milligrams per meal.

Antacids

Oral absorption of linezolid is not affected by the presence of antacids containing magnesium and aluminum hydroxide. Both drugs can safely be administered together.

Other Drugs

Some products that may interact with this drug include: Apraclonidine, atomoxetine, bethanidine, bupropion, buspirone, carbamazepine, cyclobenzaprine, dextromethorphan, certain antihistamines (azatadine, carbetapentane, chlorpheniramine), herbal products (ephedra, ginseng, tryptophan), indoramin, levodopa, maprotiline, methyldopa, certain narcotic pain relievers (fentanyl, meperidine, methadone, tapentadol), papaverine, drugs for Parkinson's disease (such as entacapone, tolcapone), rifampicin, sympathomimetics (e.g. ephedrine, methylphenidate), tetrabenazine, tricyclic antidepressants (such as amitriptyline, doxepin), other drugs which depress the bone marrow (e.g. cancer chemotherapy).

Taking other MAO inhibitors with this medication may cause a serious (possibly fatal) drug interaction. Avoid taking other MAO inhibitors (isocarboxazid, methylene blue, moclobemide, phenelzine, procarbazine, rasagiline, selegiline, tranylcypromine) during treatment with this medication. Most MAO inhibitors should also not be taken for two weeks before and after treatment with this medication.

The risk of serotonin syndrome/toxicity increases if you are also taking other drugs that increase serotonin like certain antidepressants (including mirtazapine, trazodone, SSRIs such as fluoxetine/paroxetine, SNRIs such as duloxetine/venlafaxine), tramadol, "triptans" used to treat migraine headaches (such as eletriptan, sumatriptan), tryptophan, among others. The risk of serotonin syndrome/toxicity may be more likely when you start or increase the dose of these drugs.

DRUG INTERACTIONS OF CLOFAZIMINE

Foods

Ingestion of clofazimine with orange juice resulted in a modest reduction in clofazimine bioavailability.

Antacid

Intake of aluminum-magnesium antacid produces reduction in mean bioavailability of clofazimine.

Other Drugs

May decrease absorption rate of rifampicin. Isoniazid increases clofazimine serum and urine concentrations and decreases skin concentrations.

DRUG INTERACTIONS OF CLARITHROMYCIN

Foods

Food intake immediately before dosing increases the extent of absorption by approximately 25%. However, the mean increase in metabolite area under the plasma concentration-time curve was approximately 9%.

These results suggest that clarithromycin can be taken without regard to timing in relation to meals.

Antacids

No known effect.

Other Drugs

Several cases of QT prolongation, serious ventricular arrhythmias and death have been reported due to inhibition of CYP 3A4 resulting in high blood levels of concurrently administered terfinadine/astemizole/cisapride.

IMIPENEM CILASTATIN

Other Drugs

BCG and typhoid vaccine decreases effect by pharmacological antagonism. Decreases levels of valproic acid and conjugated estrogens.

Increases levels of digoxin by altering intestinal flora. Increases ototoxicity and nephrotoxicity of tobramycin. It also decreases level of pyridoxine. Cyclosporine because of pharmacodynamic synergism increases risk of CNS toxicity.

DRUG INTERACTIONS OF BEDAQUILINE

Foods

Better absorption if taken with food, avoid alcohol.

Antacids

No known effect.

Other Drugs

Bedaquiline is metabolized by CYP3A4. Rifampicin (a CYP3A4 inducer) reduces bedaquiline in blood by half. Efavirenz based on a single dose study appears to reduce the amount of bedaquiline though inducing CYP3A4. CYP3A4 inhibitors (e.g. ciprofloxacin, erythromycin, fluconazole, clarithromycin, ketoconazole, itraconazole, ritonavir and others) can raise the level of bedaquiline but can be considered for use if the benefits outweigh the risk.

Avoid use with other drugs that prolong the QT interval as additive QT prolongation may occur (e.g. clofazimine, fluoroquinolones, delamanid, azole antifungal drugs, and many others); any syncopal event (fainting) should prompt an immediate medical evaluation and ECG.

CYP3A4 Inducers

Due to the possibility of a reduction of the therapeutic effect of bedaquiline because of the decrease in systemic exposure, coadministration of strong CYP3A4 inducers, such as rifamycins (i.e. rifampin, rifapentine and rifabutin), or moderate CYP3A4 inducers should be avoided during treatment.

CYP3A4 Inhibitors

Due to the potential risk of adverse reactions to bedaquiline because of the increase in systemic exposure, prolonged coadministration of bedaquiline and strong CYP3A4 inhibitors, such as ciprofloxacin, erythromycin, fluconazole, clarithromycin, ketoconazole, itraconazole and ritonavir (used for >14 days) should be avoided unless the benefit outweighs the risk.

Lopinavir/ritonavir

Although, clinical data in HIV/MDR-TB coinfected patients on the combined use of lopinavir (400 mg)/ritonavir (100 mg) with bedaquiline are not available, use bedaquiline with caution when coadministered with lopinavir/ritonavir and only if the benefit outweighs the risk.

Nevirapine

No dosage adjustment of bedaquiline is required when coadministered with.

Efavirenz

Concomitant administration of bedaquiline and efavirenz, or other moderate CYP3A inducers, should be avoided.

QT Interval Prolonging Drugs

Avoid use with other drugs that prolong the QT interval as additive QT prolongation may occur (e.g. clofazimine, fluoroquinolones, delamanid, azole antifungal drugs, and many others); any syncopal event (fainting) should prompt an immediate medical evaluation and ECG.

DRUG INTERACTIONS OF DELAMANID

Foods

Absorption is increased with a standard meal.

Antacids

No known effect.

Other Drugs

Avoid concomitant administration of strong CYP3A inducers (e.g. rifampicin, carbamazepine). No clinically relevant reduction in delamanid exposure was observed with weak inducers. If coadministration of delamanid with any strong inhibitor of CYP3A (e.g. ritonavir, ketokonazole) is necessary, consider more very frequent monitoring of ECGs, throughout the delamanid treatment.

Delamanid does not affect plasma exposure of coadministered anti-TB drugs, isoniazid/rifampicin/pyrazinamide/ethambutol in a clinically relevant manner (25% increases in ethambutol).

Delamanid does not affect plasma exposure of ARV drugs tenofovir, Kaletra (lopinavir/ritonavir), or efavirenz. Antiretroviral drugs, tenofovir, efavirenz, and Kaletra (lopinovir/ritonavir), do not affect delamanid exposure in a clinically relevant manner (24% increases).

Avoid using with other drugs that prolong the QT interval as additive QT prolongation may occur (e.g. clofazimine, fluoroquinolones, bedaquiline, azole antifungal drugs, ondansetron, and several others).

FURTHER READINGS

1. American Academy of Pediatrics Committee on Drugs. Transfer of drugs and other chemicals into human milk. Pediatrics. 2001;108:776-89.
2. Blumberg HM, Burman WJ, Chaisson RE, Daley CL, Etkind SC, Friedman LN, et al. American Thoracic Society/Centers for Disease Control and Prevention/Infectious Diseases Society of America: treatment of tuberculosis. Am J Respir Crit Care Med. 2003;167:603-62.
3. Caminero Luna JA. Guía de la Tuberculosis para Médicos Especialistas. Paris: Unión Internacional Contra la Tuberculosis y Enfermedades Respiratorias; 2003.
4. Companion Handbook to the WHO guidelines for the programmatic management of drug resistant tuberculosis. WHO/HTM/TB/2014.11
5. Cynamon MH, Klemens SP, et al. Activity of several novel oxazolidinones against mycobacterium tuberculosis in a murinemodel. Antimicrob. Agents Chemother. 1999;43:1189-91.
6. Guidelines for programmatic management of drug resistant tuberculosis. WHO, 2011. WHO/HTM/TB/2011.6
7. Handbook of Anti-Tuberculosis Agents. Tuberculosis (Edinb). 2008;88:100-1.
8. Jagannath C, Venkta Reddy M, et al. Chemotheraputic activity of Clofazimine and its analoge against m.tuberculosis in vitro and in vivo. Am J Respir Crit Care Med. 1995;151:1083-6.
9. Jones RN, Jhonson DM, et al. In vitro antimicrobial activity and spectra of U-100592 and U100766. The two novel fluorinated oxazolidine group. Antimicrob.Agents Chemother. 1996;40:720-6.
10. Lehman J. Paraaminosalicylic acid in treatment of tuberculosis. Lancet 1946;1:15-6.
11. Malone RS, Fish DN, Spiegel DM, Childs JM, Peloquin CA. The effect of hemodialysis on cycloserine, ethionamide, para-aminosalicylate, and clofazimine. Chest. 1999;116:984-90.

12. Ministério da Saúde. Secretaria de Vigilância em Saúde. Centro de Referência Prof. Hélio Fraga. Tuberculose Multirresistente: Guia de Vigilância Epidemiológica. Rio de Janeiro: Centro de Referência Professor Hélio Fraga/SVS/Ministério da Saúde e Projeto MSH; 2007.
13. O'Donnell JA, Gelone SP. Fluoroquinolones. Infect Dis Clin North Am. 2000;14:489-513, xi.
14. Para-aminosalicylic acid. Tuberculosis (Edinb). 2008;88:137-8.
15. Tsukamura M, Nakamura E, et al. Theraputic effect of new anti bacterial substance Ofloxacin. Am Rev Respir Dis. 1987;136:1339-42.
16. WHO treatment guidelines for Drug-Resistent Tuberculosis – 2016 Update. WHO/HTM/TB/2016.04.
17. World Health Organization. Guidelines for the Programmatic Management of Drug-Resistant Tuberculosis: Emergency Update 2008. Geneva: World Health Organization, Stop TB Department; 2008.
18. World Health Organization. Treatment of Tuberculosis: Guidelines, 4th edition. Geneva: World Health Organization; 2009.

CHAPTER

Interactions between Anti-tubercular Drugs Used in New Patients with Foods and Drugs

ISONIAZID

Foods/Drugs	Interactions
Foods	Decreases absorption of isoniazid, isoniazid usually taken on empty stomach
Cheese and red wine	Inhibition of monoamine oxidase enzyme and should not be taken concomitantly with Isoniazid
Fish	Increases concentration of histamine
Antacid/ Aluminium hydroxide/ Ranitidine	Decreases absorption of isoniazid and should be administered one hour after Isoniazid
Valproic acid	Increases serum concentration of valproic acid
Oral anticoagulants	Increases serum concentration of the anticoagulant
Benzodiazepines	Increases serum concentration of benzodiazepines
Enflurane	Possibility of nephrotoxicity
Carbamazepine	Increases serum concentration of carbamazepine
Corticosteroids	Decreases serum levels of isoniazid
Ketoconazole	Decreases serum concentration of ketoconazole
Cycloserine	Greater neurotoxicity
Diazepam	Increases serum concentration of diazepam
Disulfiram	Increases possibility of psychotic events
Phenytoin	Increases serum concentration of phenytoin
Levodopa	Increases serum concentration of catecholamines
Paracetamol	Greater hepatotoxicity
Rifampicin	Greater hepatotoxicity
Theophylline	Increases concentration of theophylline

RIFAMPICIN

Foods/Drugs	Interactions
Foods	Decreases absorption of rifampicin. Rifampicin should be taken on empty stomach, usually 45 minutes before breakfast
Antacids containing aluminium hydroxide	Can delay the absorption of rifampicin

(Contd.)

(Contd.)

Foods/Drugs	Interactions
Para-aminosalicylic acid	Decreases absorption of rifampicin
Amiodarone	Decreases serum levels of amiodarone
Oral anticoagulants	Decreases serum levels of anticoagulant
Contraceptives	Decreases serum levels of contraceptives. Advised to switch over to an oral contraceptive containing higher dose (50 μg) of estrogen or use alternative method of contraception
Anticonvulsants	Decreases serum levels of anticonvulsants
Tricyclic antidepressants	Decreases serum levels of antidepressants
Antipsychotics	Decreases serum levels of antipsychotics
Barbiturates and benzodiazepines	Decreases serum levels of barbiturates and benzodiazepines
Beta blocker	Decreases serum levels of beta blocker
Cyclosporine	Reduce effect of cyclosporine
Ketoconazole	Decreases serum levels of ketoconazole
Codeine	Decreases serum levels of codeine
Corticosteroids	Decreases serum levels of corticosteroids
Dapsone	May decrease the serum levels of dapsone
Digoxin	Decreases serum levels of digoxin
Diltiazem	Decreases serum levels of diltiazem
Enalapril	Decreases serum levels of enalapril
Statins	Decreases serum levels of statins
Fluconazole	Decreases serum levels of fluconazole
Haloperidol	Decreases serum levels of haloperidol
Oral hypoglycemic agents	Decreases serum levels of hypoglycemic agents Dose of hypoglycemic agents might have to be increased
Itraconazole	Decreases serum levels of itraconazole
Methadone	Decreases serum levels of methadone
Morphine	Decreases serum levels of morphine
Narcotics and analgesics	Decreases serum levels of narcotics and analgesics
Propafenone	Decreases serum levels of propafenone
Nifedipine	Decreases serum levels of nifedipine
Quinidine	Decreases serum levels of quinidine
Theophylline	Decreases serum levels of theophylline
Verapamil	Decreases serum levels of verapamil
Isoniazid + ketoconazole	Greater hepatotoxicity
Ethionamide	Greater hepatotoxicity
Phenytoin	Greater hepatotoxicity
Isoniazid	Greater hepatotoxicity
Sulfonamides	Greater hepatotoxicity
Pyrazinamide	Greater uric acid excretion
Efavirenz	Decreases serum levels of efavirenz
Indinavir	Decreases serum levels of indinavir
Lopinavir/ritonavir	Decreases serum levels of lopinavir
Nelfinavir	Decreases serum levels of nelfinavir
Saquinavir	Decreases serum levels of saquinavir
Zidovudine	Decreases serum levels of zidovudine

PYRAZINAMIDE

Foods/Drugs	Interactions
Foods	Little impact on absorption of pyrazinamide
Antacids	No interference with the absorption of pyrazinamide
Allopurinol	Decreases effect of allopurinol, pyrazinamide Increases the serum levels of uric acid
Colchicine	Decreases effect of colchicines, pyrazinamide Increases the serum levels of uric acid
Cyclosporine	Decreases serum concentration of cyclosporine
Ketoconazole	Greater hepatotoxicity
Ethionamide	The adverse effect of ethionamide can increase
Rifampicin	Greater hepatotoxicity
Isoniazid	Greater hepatotoxicity

ETHAMBUTOL

Foods/Drugs	Interactions
Foods	No impact on bioavailability of ethambutol
Antacids	Decreased absorption of ethambutol and should be administered at longer intervals
Ethionamide	Increased possibility of nephrotoxicity
Ethacrynic acid	Increased possibility of ototoxicity
Amphotericin	Increases possibility of nephrotoxicity

FURTHER READINGS

1. Baciewicz AM, Chrisman CR, Finch CK, Self TH. Update on rifampicin and rifabutin drug interactions. Am J Med Sci. 2008;335:126-36.
2. Blumberg HM, Burman WJ, Chaisson RE, Daley CL, Etkind SC, Friedman LN, et al. American Thoracic Society/Centers for Disease Control and Prevention/Infectious Diseases Society of America: treatment of tuberculosis. Am J Respir Crit Care Med. 2003;167:603-62.
3. Caminero Luna JA. Guía de la Tuberculosis para Médicos Especialistas. Paris: Unión Internacional Contra la Tuberculosis y Enfermedades Respiratorias; 2003.
4. Chemotherapy and management of tuberculosis in the United Kingdom: recommendations 1998. Joint Tuberculosis Committee of the British Thoracic Society. Thorax. 1998;53:536-48.
5. Desta Z, Soukhova NV, Flockhart DA. Inhibition of cytochrome P450 (CYP450) isoforms by isoniazid: potent inhibition of CYP2C19 and CYP3A. Antimicrob Agents Chemother. 2001;45:382-92.
6. Dooley KE, Chaisson RE. Tuberculosis and diabetes mellitus: convergence of two epidemics. Lancet Infect Dis. 2009;9:737-46.
7. Engelhard D, Stutman HR, Marks MI. Interaction of ketoconazole with rifampicin and isoniazid. N Engl J Med. 1984;311:1681-3.
8. Migliori GB, D'Arcy Richardson M, Sotgiu G, Lange C. Multidrug-resistant and extensively drug-resistant tuberculosis in the West. Europe and United States: epidemiology, surveillance, and control. Clin Chest Med. 2009;30:637-65, vii.
9. Nahid P, et al. ATS/CDC/IDSA Clinical Practice Guidelines: Treatment of Drug-Susceptible Tuberculosis. Clin Infec Dis 2016:1-50.
10. Niemi M, Backman JT, Fromm MF, Neuvonen PJ, Kivistö KT. Pharmacokinetic interactions with rifampicin: clinical relevance. Clin Pharmacokinet. 2003;42:819 50.

11. Pai MP, Momary KM, Rodvold KA. Antibiotic drug interactions. Med Clin North Am. 2006;90:1223-55.
12. Self TH, Chrisman CR, Baciewicz AM, Bronze MS. Isoniazid drug and food interactions. Am J Med Sci. 1999;317:304-11.
13. Technical and Operational Guidelines for TB Control in India 2016.
14. World Health Organization. Treatment of TB Guidelines - 4th edition. WHO/HTM/TB/2009.420
15. World Health Organization. Treatment of Tuberculosis: Guidelines for National Programmes. Geneva: World Health Organization; 2003.
16. Yew WW. Clinically significant interactions with drugs used in the treatment of tuberculosis. Drug Saf. 2002;25:111-33.

CHAPTER 10

Interactions between Antitubercular Drugs Used in Drug Resistant Patients with Foods and Drugs

AMINOGLYCOSIDES (STREPTOMYCIN, KANAMYCIN, AMIKACIN)

Foods/Drugs	Interactions
Acyclovir	Increased possibility of nephrotoxicity
Ethacrynic acid	Increased possibility of ototoxicity
Amphotericin	Increased possibility of nephrotoxicity
Oral anticoagulant	Greater effect of the anticoagulant
Nonsteroidal anti-inflammatory drugs	Increased possibility of ototoxicity and nephrotoxicity
Capreomycin	Increased possibility of ototoxicity and nephrotoxicity
Cephalosporins	Increased possibility of nephrotoxicity
Cisplatin	Increased possibility of nephrotoxicity
Cyclosporine	Increased possibility of nephrotoxicity
Furosemide	Increased possibility of ototoxicity
Methotrexate	Possible increase in the toxicity of methotrexate
Polymyxins	Greater nephrotoxicity
Vancomycin	Greater ototoxicity and nephrotoxicity
Neuromuscular blocking agents	Additive effect
Thiacetazone	Greater ototoxicity of streptomycin

CAPREOMYCIN

Foods/Drugs	Interactions
Neuromuscular blocking agents	Increases adverse effects of the two drugs
Aminoglycosides	Increases adverse effects of the two drugs
Polymyxin B	Increases adverse effects of the two drugs

FLUOROQUINOLONES

Foods/Drugs	Interactions
Foods	No effect
Dairy products with high concentration of calcium	Interfere with absorption of fluoroquinolones
Antacids with cations Ca, Mg, Al and Fe	Decreases absorption of fluoroquinolones
Sucralfate	Decreases absorption of fluoroquinolone

(Contd.)

(Contd.)

Foods/Drugs	Interactions
Drugs metabolized by cytochrome P450: cyclosporine, theophylline, warfarin, phenytoin and sulfonylurea	Increases effect of these drugs
Nonsteroidal anti-inflammatory drugs	Increases stimulation of the central nervous system and possibility of convulsions
Probenecid	Increases serum levels of the fluoroquinolones
Theophylline	Increases serum levels of theophylline

ETHIONAMIDE/PROTHIONAMIDE

Foods/Drugs	Interactions
Foods	Minimal effect on bioavailability of ethionamide
Antacid	Do not interfere with absorption of ethionamide
Alcohol	Increased possibility of psychotic reactions
Isoniazid	Temporarily increases serum concentration of isoniazid
Para-aminosalicylic acid	Increases possibility of hypothyroidism
Cycloserine/terizidone	Increases possibility of toxic effects on the central nervous system
Dapsone	Potentiates peripheral neuritis

CYCLOSERINE/TERIZIDONE

Foods/Drugs	Interactions
Foods	Decrease and delay in absorption of cycloserine/terizidone
Orange juice and other acidic beverages	Decrease concentration of cycloserine/terizidone, drug should be ingested with water well before or after meals
Antacid	No effect on absorption of cycloserine/terizidone
Alcohol	Increases effects of alcohol and dizziness
Anticoagulants	Increases serum concentration of the anticoagulants
Ethionamide	Possibility of increased toxic effects on the central nervous system
Phenytoin	Increases serum concentration of phenytoin
Isoniazid	Possibility of increased toxic effects on the central nervous system
Vitamin B6	Increases vitamin B6 clearance

PARA-AMINOSALICYLIC ACID(PAS)

Foods/Drugs	Interactions
Foods	Increase the absorption of PAS. Drug is administered with water, orange juice or fatty foods
Antacid	No effect on absorption of PAS
Anticoagulants	Possibility of increased anticoagulant effect
Digoxin	Decreases serum levels of digoxin

(Contd.)

(Contd.)

Foods/Drugs	Interactions
Corticosteroids	Possibility of adverse effects of the corticosteroids
Ethionamide	Increased possibility of hypothyroidism and hepatotoxicity
Isoniazid	Possibility of increased serum levels of isoniazid
Probenecid	Increases serum concentration of para-aminosalicylic acid
Vitamin B12	Decreases levels of vitamin B12
Sulfonylurea	Possibility of increased hypoglycemic effects of sulfonylurea

LINEZOLID

Foods/Drugs	Interactions
Foods with higher tyramine content like stored meat, fish, dairy products, aged cheese, soya sauce, tap beers, red wines	Avoid food or drinks with high tyramine content, may cause serious rise in blood pressure
Antacids	No effect on absorption of linezolid
MAO inhibitors	Serious (possible fatal) drug interaction
Antidepressants including mirtazapine, trazodone, SSRIs such as fluoxetine/paroxetine, SNRIs such as duloxetine/venlafaxine	Serotonin syndrome/toxicity increases
Tramadol, "triptans" used to treat migraine headaches (such as eletriptan, sumatriptan), tryptophan, among others	Serotonin syndrome/toxicity increases

CLOFAZIMINE

Foods/Drugs	Interactions
High fatty meal	Increases bioavailability
Orange juice	Reduction in bioavailability of clofazimine
Antacid (aluminum-magnesium)	Decreases bioavailability of clofazimine
Rifampicin	Decreases rifampicin absorption
Isoniazid	Increases clofazimine serum and urine concentrations and decreases skin concentrations
Sodium picosulfate/magnesium antioxidants/anhydrous citric acid	Decreases effect of clofazimine

CLARITHROMYCIN

Foods/Drugs	Interactions
Foods	Increases the absorption of clarithromycin
Antacid	Decreases the absorption of clarithromycin
Amphotericin B	Increases nephrotoxicity and ototoxicity
Acyclovir, Adefovir, Amikacin, Carboplatin, Cyclosporine, Gentamicin, Kanamycin, Tobramycin	Increases nephrotoxicity and ototoxicity
Streptomycin, Pentamidine, Vancomycin	Increases nephrotoxicity and ototoxicity
Atracurium, Pancuronium, Rocuronium	Pharmacodynamic Synergism
Terfinadine/astemizole/cisapride	QT prolongation, serious ventricular arrhythmias and death due to high blood level of terfinadine/astemizole/cisapride

IMIPENEM CILASTATIN

Foods/Drugs	Interactions
BCG and typhoid vaccine	Decreases effect of BCG and typhoid vaccine by pharmalogical antagonism
Valproic acid	Decreases levels valproic acid
Conjugated estrogens	Decreases levels conjugated estrogens
Digoxin	Increases levels of digoxin by altering intestinal flora
Tobramycin	Increases ototoxicity and nephrotoxicity of tobramycin
Pyridoxine	Decreases level of pyridoxine
Cyclosporine	Pharmacodynamic synergism increases risk of CNS toxicity

AMOXYCLAV

Foods/Drugs	Interactions
Foods	No effect, usualy taken at the start of meal to enhance absorption of amoxicillin and to minimize GI intolerance
High fat meals	Decreases the absorption of clavulanate
Antacids	No effect
Probenecid	Increased and prolonged blood concentration of amoxicillin
Oral anticoagulants	Abnormal prolongation of prothrombin time Appropriate monitoring and adjustment of dose of anticoagulants
Allopurinol	Increase in incidence of rashes
Oral contraceptives	Decreases estrogen reabsorption and reduce efficacy of oral contraceptives

BEDAQUILINE

Foods/Drugs	Interactions
Foods	Better absorption if taken with food
Alcohol	Avoid
Rifampicin	Decreases dose in blood by half
Efavirenz	Reduces amount
Azole antifungals agents(ketoconazole, itraconazole)	Raise level, additive QT prolongation
Macrolides	Raise level
Protease inhibitors	Raise level
Clofazimine	Additive QT prolongation
Fluoroquinolones	Additive QT prolongation
Delamanid	Additive QT prolongation

DELAMANID

Foods/Drugs	Interactions
Foods	Better absorption if taken with food
Rifampicin	Decreases level
Carbamazepine	Decreases level
Efavirenz	Reduces amount
Ritonavir	Additive QT prolongation
Clofazimine	Additive QT prolongation
Fluoroquinolones	Additive QT prolongation
Bedaquiline	Additive QT prolongation
Azole antifungal drugs	Additive QT prolongation
Ondansetron	Additive QT prolongation

FURTHER READINGS

1. American Academy of Pediatrics Committee on Drugs. Transfer of drugs and other chemicals into human milk. Pediatrics. 2001;108:776-89.
2. Blumberg HM, Burman WJ, Chaisson RE, Daley CL, Etkind SC, Friedman LN, et al. American Thoracic Society/Centers for Disease Control and Prevention/Infectious Diseases Society of America: treatment of tuberculosis. Am J Respir Crit Care Med. 2003;167:603-62.
3. Caminero Luna JA. Guía de la Tuberculosis para Médicos Especialistas. Paris: Unión Internacional Contra la Tuberculosis y Enfermedades Respiratorias; 2003.
4. Companion Handbook to the WHO guidelines for the programmatic management of drug resistant tuberculosis. WHO/HTM/TB/2014.11
5. Companion Handbook to the WHO guidelines for the programmatic management of drug resistant tuberculosis. WHO/HTM/TB/2014.11.
6. Cynamon MH, Klemens SP, et al. Activity of several novel oxazolidinones against mycobacterium tuberculosis in a murinemodel. Antimicrob, Agents Chemother. 1999, 43:1189-91.
7. Guidelines for programmatic management of drug resistant tuberculosis. WHO, 2011. WHO/HTM/TB/2011.6
8. Handbook of Anti-Tuberculosis Agents. Tuberculosis (Edinb). 2008;88:100-1.

9. Jagannath C, Venkta Reddy M, et al. Chemotheraputic activity of Clofazimine and its analoge against m.tuberculosis in vitro and in vivo. Am J Respir Crit Care Med. 1995;151:1083-6.
10. Jones RN, Jhonson DM, et al. In vitro antimicrobial activity and spectra of U-100592 and U100766. The two novel fluorinated oxazolidine group. Antimicrob Agents Chemother. 1996, 40:720-6.
11. Lehman J. Paraaminosalicylic acid in treatment of tuberculosis. Lancet. 1946; 1:15-6.
12. Malone RS, Fish DN, Spiegel DM, Childs JM, Peloquin CA. The effect of hemodialysis on cycloserine, ethionamide, para-aminosalicylate, and clofazimine. Chest. 1999;116:984-90.
13. Ministério da Saúde. Secretaria de Vigilância em Saúde. Centro de Referência Prof. Hélio Fraga. Tuberculose Multirresistente: Guia de Vigilância Epidemiológica. Rio de Janeiro: Centro de Referência Professor Hélio Fraga/SVS/Ministério da Saúde e Projeto MSH; 2007.
14. O'Donnell JA, Gelone SP. Fluoroquinolones. Infect Dis Clin North Am. 2000;14:489-513, xi.
15. Para-aminosalicylic acid. Tuberculosis (Edinb). 2008;88:137-8.
16. Technical and Operational Guidelines for TB Control in India 2016.
17. Tsukamura M, Nakamura E, et al. Theraputic effect of new anti bacterial substance Ofloxacin. Am Rev Respir Dis. 1987;136:1339-42.
18. WHO treatment guidelines for Drug-Resistent Tuberculosis – 2016 Update. WHO/HTM/TB/2016.04.
19. World Health Organization. Guidelines for the Programmatic Management of Drug-Resistant Tuberculosis: Emergency Update 2008. Geneva: World Health Organization, Stop TB Department; 2008.
20. World Health Organization. Treatment of Tuberculosis: Guidelines. 4th ed. Geneva: World Health Organization; 2009.

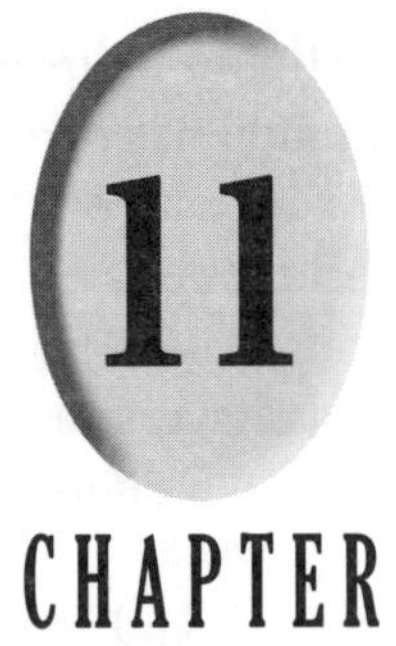

CHAPTER

Treatment of Tuberculosis in Pregnancy, Renal Insufficiency and Liver Diseases

Treatment of tuberculosis poses a difficult clinical problem in special situations like pregnancy, renal insufficiency and liver diseases. There are various concerns regarding dosage, toxicity and way of administration.

TREATMENT OF TUBERCULOSIS IN PREGNANCY AND LACTATION

Isoniazid is considered safe in pregnancy, except for some chance of postpartum hepatitis. American Thoracic Society (ATS) recommends supplementation of pyridoxine during pregnancy (25 mg/day). Use of rifampicin and ethambutol is safe in pregnancy. Data regarding other rifamycins (rifabutin and rifapentine) is insufficient, and thus they should be cautiously used. Safety regarding pyrazinamide could not be assured, but World Health Organization (WHO) and International Union against Tuberculosis and Lung Disease (IUATLD) recommend its use in pregnancy, because when used for 6 months regimen benefits may outweigh possible risk.

Streptomycin may cause congenital deafness, as this drug interferes with development of ear. Other injectables, like amikacin, kanamycin and capreomycin having pharmacokinetics similar to streptomycin, may also cause fetal nephrotoxicity and ototoxicity. Ethionamide and prothionamide are contraindicated in pregnancy, as they are found teratogenic in animal studies. Cycloserine crosses placenta, and since its safety in pregnancy is not established, it should be avoided, and used only if no other suitable alternatives are available. PAS has been used safely in pregnancy in past, but since no well designed study has been done to ascertain its safety in pregnancy, it should be used in absence of any other alternative. Flouroquinolones being toxic and inhibitor of growing cartilage in animals, is to be avoided in pregnancy. Animal studies demonstrated teratogenicity (retardation of fetal skull ossification) for clofazimine and crossing of placenta and excretion in milk. However, WHO has approved this drug safe in pregnancy. Similarly, clarithromycin is not safe in pregnancy as higher dose has been associated with embryotoxicity. There are no adequate and well controlled studies regarding teratogenecity of linezolid in pregnant women. It should be used during pregnancy only if the potential benefit justifies the potential risk to the fetus. Bedaquiline is not recommended during pregnancy or breastfeeding due to limited data. Reproduction studies performed in rats and rabbits have revealed no evidence of harm to the fetus. There are very limited data from the use of delamanid in pregnant women. Studies in animals have shown reproductive toxicity. Available pharmacokinetic data in animals have shown excretion of delamanid and/or its metabolites in milk.

Regarding treatment of tuberculosis in a pregnant lady it is said that, treatment of tuberculosis is far less hazardous than leaving the disease untreated, both with regard to baby and mother. Tuberculosis in pregnant lady may lead to underweight infant or congenital tuberculosis. Risk of miscarriage is much higher in active tuberculosis than risk from the drug treatment, so standard treatment should be given. Treatment regimen for drug sensitive tuberculosis should include rifampicin, isoniazid and ethambutol. Streptomycin should not be used. Opinion regarding use of pyrazinamide is divided, but WHO and IUATLD recommend its use. ATS does not confidently advocate it. According to WHO, 6 month regimen based upon isoniazid, rifampicin and pyrazinamide should be used whenever possible, and ethambutol should be used if a fourth drug is needed during initial phase. Contrary to this, ATS recommends that pyrazinamide should better be avoided in pregnancy, because of lack of sufficient data for its safety. If pyrazinamide is not used, duration of treatment should be 9 months. Although isoniazid, rifampicin and ethambutol cross the placenta, are not found to be teratogenic.

Women taking first line antitubercular drugs should not be asked for termination of pregnancy, while those on reserve line drugs should be counseled for possible adverse effects. Breastfeeding should not be discouraged, as amount secreted in milk is insufficient to cause any toxic or therapeutic effect. Supplemental pyridoxine is recommended for both nursing mother and her infant, even if no isoniazid is being given to the infant. All antitubercular drugs could be used during lactation, except flouroquinolones because of possible risk. Baby of woman who has taken rifampicin during pregnancy should receive vitamin K at birth, to avoid the risk of postnatal hemorrhage, as rifampicin may induce metabolism of vitamin K and hamper hepatic synthesis of vitamin K dependent coagulation factors.

Women taking oral hormonal contraceptives, should be counselled for possible contraceptive failure and occurrence of pregnancy, especially in rifampicin containing antitubercular treatment regimen, because of induction of metabolism of contraceptive drug by rifampicin. Such ladies should be advised to use non-hormonal contraceptive during, and for one month after treatment with rifampicin containing regimen.

TREATMENT OF TB IN RENAL INSUFFICIENCY

Treatment of tuberculosis in renal insufficiency poses a difficult clinical problem, because various antituberculosis medications are cleared by kidney. On one side it raises concern of drug-induced toxicity, due to impaired excretion by diseased kidney, while on the other side, it raises concern of under treatment of tuberculosis. In later situation, adequate peak serum concentration is usually low, and not of therapeutic use. Another issue of concern is the therapeutic level of antitubercular drugs in patients with end-stage renal disease, undergoing hemodialysis, which clears some drugs easily, than others.

TABLE 11.1: Dosing recommendation for adult patients with renal insufficiency or undergoing hemodialysis.

Drug	Change in frequency	Dose and frequency in patients with creatinine clearance <30 mL/min or those on hemodialysis.
Isoniazid	No change needed	300 mg daily or 900 mg thrice a week
Rifampicin	No change needed	600 mg daily or 600 mg thrice a week
Pyrazinamide	Yes	25–35 mg/kg per dose three times a week
Ethambutol	Yes	15–25 mg/kg per dose three times a week
Rifabutin	No	Normal dose can be used, if possible monitor drug concentrations to avoid toxicity
Rifapentine	No	No adjustment necessary
Levofloxacin	Yes	750–1000 mg per dose three times a week
Moxifloxacin	No	No adjustment necessary
Gatifloxacin	No	400 mg three times a week
Ofloxacin	Yes	600–800 mg per dose three times per week
Cycloserine	Yes	250 mg daily or 500 mg three times a week
Terizidone		Recommendations not available
Ethionamide	No change needed	250–500 mg daily
PAS	No change needed	4 g/dose twice daily
Streptomycin	Yes	12–15 mg/kg/dose twice or three times a week
Capreomycin	Yes	12–15 mg/kg/dose twice or three times a week
Kanamycin	Yes	12–15 mg/kg/dose twice or three times a week
Amikacin	Yes	12–15 mg/kg/dose twice or three times a week
Clarithromycin	Yes	Usual dose 500 mg twice daily but can be reduced to 250 mg twice daily
Linezolid	No change needed	Usual dose is 600 mg twice daily but can be reduced to 600 mg once daily after 4–6 weeks
Clofazimine	Yes	Begin with 300 mg daily and decreased to 100 mg daily after 4–6 weeks

Contd...

Contd...

Drug	Change in frequency	Dose and frequency in patients with creatinine clearance <30 mL/min or those on hemodialysis.
Amoxicillin and clavulanic acid	Yes	Dose used is 625 mg twice daily, 1000 mg should not be used
Bedaquiline	No	No dosage adjustment is required in patients with mild to moderate renal impairment (dosing not established in severe renal impairment, use with caution)
Delamanid	No	No dosage adjustment is required in patients with mild to moderate renal impairment (dosing not established in severe renal impairment, use with caution)
Imipenem/ cilastatin	Yes	For creatinine clearance 20–40 mL/min dose 500 mg every 8 hours; for creatinine clearance <20 mL/min dose 500 mg every 12 hours
Meropenem	Yes	For creatinine clearance 20–40 mL/min dose 750 mg every 12 hours; for creatinine clearance <20 mL/min dose 500 mg every 12 hours
High dose isoniazid		Recommendations not available

British Thoracic Society, advocates dose reduction for drugs which are excreted by renal route, while American Thoracic Society prefers increasing the dosing interval instead of decreasing the dose. Administration of drugs which are excreted by kidney should be changed by increasing the dosing interval, if creatinine clearance falls below 30 mL/min (Table 11.1). There is paucity of data to guide the dosing recommendation if creatinine clearance is above 30 mL/min, when standard doses should be prescribed. Rifampicin and isoniazid are eliminated by liver, and they could be given in usual dose. Population with slow hepatic acetylation of isoniazid could be given supplemental pyridoxine to prevent peripheral neuropathy. Alteration in dose of ethambutol which is 80% excreted by kidney, should be made if creatinine clearance falls below 70 mL/min, to lowest possible dose, but if it falls below 30 mL/min. It should be given intermittently as three times a week in dose of 15-20 mg/kg body weight. Pyrazinamide is metabolized in liver, but its metabolites, pyrazinoic acid and 5-hydroxypyrazinoic acid are excreted by kidney and thus drug should be given three times a week, in dose of 25-35 mg/kg body weight, to avoid toxicity, if creatinine clearance falls below 30 mL/min (Table 11.1). Apart from this, risk of developing hyperuricemia with pyrazinamide is increased in cases of renal insufficiency. Since streptomycin is predominantly excreted by renal route, and removed by hemodialysis to a significant extent (about 40%), it should be administered three times a week in dose of 12-15 mg/kg body weight (Table 11.1) in patients of renal insufficiency with creatinine clearance below 30 mL/min, and those on hemodialysis. Since, pharmacokinetics of other aminoglycosides is similar to streptomycin, they need similar modification of dose. Renal clearance of fluoroquinolones varies from drug to drug. It is greater for levofloxacin than moxifloxacin. Dose adjustment for fluroquinolones is recommended if creatinine clearance is less than 30 mL/min (750–1000 mg three times a week) ethionamide need no or little alteration of administration as it is not excreted by kidney but, if creatinine clearance is less than 30 mL/min, dose of ethionamide should be reduced to 250–500 mg/day (Table 11.1). Dose of cycloserine should be modified if creatinine clearance falls below 30 mL/min or patient is on hemodialysis. It should be changed to 500 mg thrice a week or 250 mg daily (Table 11.1); evidence for safety of 250 mg daily dose of cycloserine is not yet established with regard to neuropathy, and 500 mg three times a week, is preferred in this regard. Serum concentrations of drug should be monitored. PAS is not safe in renal disease and should only be given if no other alternative are available, as it may aggravate metabolic acidosis. If it is to be given, it should be given at dose of 4 g/dose, twice daily. Thioacetazone being excreted in urine, it should not be given to patients with renal disease. The pharmacokinetics of the parent drug, linezolid, are not altered in patients with any degree of renal insufficiency but metabolites of linezolid may accumulate in patients with renal insufficiency, with the amount of accumulation increasing with the severity of renal dysfunction. Therefore, no dose adjustment is recommended for patients with renal insufficiency. However, given the absence of information on the clinical significance of accumulation of the primary metabolites, use of linezolid in patients with renal insufficiency should be weighed against the potential risks of accumulation of these metabolites. Clofazimine is safe in patients having renal disease as excretion is mainly through biliary route. In patients with severe renal impairment dose of clarithromycin must be reduced. Imipenem is highly nephrotoxic but addition of cilastatin lessens its toxicity. No dosage adjustment is required in patients with mild to moderate renal impairment with bedaquiline (dosing not established in severe renal impairment, use with caution). No dosage adjustment is required in patients with mild to moderate renal impairment with delamanid. Dosing not established in severe renal impairment, use with caution and only when the benefits outweigh the risks.

Hemodialysis removes the drug before its therapeutic effect, but if the drug is given sufficient time before hemodialysis, so that it gets time to be distributed throughout the body, far less drug is likely to be removed. Administration of drug after hemodialysis, will avoid premature removal of drug on one hand, and facilitate Directly Observed Treatment Short Course (DOTS) on the other hand. Premature removal of second line drugs, by hemodialysis, may further aggravate the problem of drug resistance by exposing the tubercle *bacillus* to subtherapeutic drug concentration.

Rifampicin, isoniazid and ethambutol are removed to insignificant extent by hemodialysis, but pyrazinamide is removed to a significant extent. Thus supplemental dosing is not needed with isoniazid, rifampicin and ethambutol, in patients of end stage renal disease, undergoing hemodialysis. Similar to streptomycin, about 40% of drugs like kanamycin, amikacin and capreomycin are removed from blood, if they are given just before hemodialysis. Flouroquinolone and ethionamide are not cleared by hemodialysis and thus their dose need not be altered in this situation. Usually hemodialysis does not pose significant problem, if drugs are given after the procedure.

Ideally, it is important to monitor serum concentrations of drugs in persons with renal failure who are taking aminoglycosides, cycloserine or ethambutol to provide effective therapeutic drug concentration and also to minimize dose-related toxicity. Patients with renal failure may have other comorbid conditions, like diabetes mellitus and gastroparesis, which may further complicate the pharmacokinetics of drugs. Presently, there is no data to guide administration of antitubercular drug use in patients undergoing peritoneal dialysis, and for this subset of patients, recommendations of hemodialysis are applicable. The safest regimen that is being advised in patients diagnosed as new cases of tuberculosis with renal insufficiency, is rifampicin, isoniazid and pyrazinamide for two months followed by rifampicin and isoniazid for next four months.

TREATMENT OF TB IN LIVER DISEASES

Treatment of tuberculosis, with deranged liver functions presents with two major clinical scenarios. First is use of antitubercular drugs in persons with pre-existing liver disease, and second is antitubercular drug-induced hepatotoxicity. Various antitubercular drugs are potentially hepatotoxic, and administration of these drugs may aggravate liver disease, in a patient with compromised liver function. Drugs like ethambutol, streptomycin, kanamycin, amikacin and capreomycin are safe in liver disease as they are neither significantly metabolized, nor toxic to liver.

Drug-induced Hepatotoxicity

It is found that, period of latency between start of drug regimen and occurrence of drug induced hepatitis is usually four to nine days. It must be known that, about 10–30% of patients receiving antitubercular therapy may normally have transient rise of bilirubin and liver enzymes serum glutarylpyruvate transaminase (SGPT) and serum glutaryloxalate transaminase (SGOT), to about 1 to 3 times the normal, during first two months of therapy, which comes down on continuation of treatment. It is of interest to note that about 10% of patients, who develop mild transaminase elevation (i.e. 1–2% of all adults treated) may have severe hepatitis and liver failure until the drug is discontinued. This clinical condition has case fatality of approximately 10%. Drug-induced hepatitis is considered, when serum level of SGPT or SGOT rises more than 150 IU/L on more than three occasions, or greater than 250 IU/L on one occasion, along with values of serum bilirubin more than 34.2 micromol/lit (2 mg%).

Data indicate that incidence of isoniazid induced, clinical hepatitis is lesser than was previously thought. Hepatitis occurs in 0.6% patients, if isoniazid is given alone, but incidence is 1.6% if it is given with drugs, other than rifampicin. With rifampicin, incidence of hepatitis is 2.7%. Risk of drug-induced hepatitis, increases with age, and it is 2% in persons aged 50–64 years. Rate of fatal hepatitis is 0.023%. If it is given to patient with pre-existing liver disease, it may accumulate in body and further increases risk of drug-induced hepatitis. Frequent monitoring of serum level of hepatic transaminases is indicated in this clinical setting.

Patients with alcoholic liver disease, are at increased risk of peripheral neuropathy, and should be given pyridoxine prophylactically at dose of 10 mg daily. Rifampicin may cause normal transient hyperbilirubinemia in 0.6% patients. Incidence of hepatitis is 2.7% if it is given with isoniazid, and it is 1.1%, if given with drug other than isoniazid. Clearance of rifampicin, may be impaired, causing serum levels to rise, if it is given to patient with pre-existing liver disease. Careful monitoring of liver functions is indicated in these patients.

The first-line drugs isoniazid, rifampicin and pyrazinamide are all associated with hepatotoxicity. Of the three, rifampicin is least likely to cause hepatocellular damage, although it is associated with cholestatic jaundice. Pyrazinamide is the most hepatotoxic of the three first-line drugs. Among the second-line drugs, ethionamide, prothionamide and para-aminosalicylic acid (PAS) can also be hepatotoxic, although less so than any of the first-line drugs. Hepatitis occurs rarely with the fluoroquinolones.

Chemical structure of ethionamide is similar to isoniazid, and it can cause liver toxicity in about 2% patients, and should be cautiously used in pre-existing liver disease. PAS may cause clinical hepatitis in 0.3% cases. Since, pharmacokinetics of PAS is not significantly altered in liver disease, it could be used in usual doses and usual regimen. Cycloserine could be safely used in liver disease, except in case of alcohol related hepatitis, where it increases risk of seizures. Thioacetazone is hepatotoxic, and it should be avoided. Fluoroquinolones except ciprofloxacin are safe for use in liver disease.

Advanced age, female sex, poor nutritional status, pre-existing liver disease, chronic alcoholism, Hepatitis B carrier state and slow acetylator status, are considered risk factors for antitubercular drug-induced hepatitis. Several studies have observed relation between serum markers for viral hepatitis and antitubercular drug-induced hepatitis. It has been observed, that viral hepatitis complicates treatment more frequently with regimen containing both rifampicin and isoniazid, than in regimen having only one of them or none of them.

It is often difficult to find the culprit drug, in a multidrug regimen, causing drug-induced hepatitis. Regarding this practical problem, it is said that, rise in serum transaminase activity within 15 days of starting regimen, is usually attributed to rifampicin, but if it occurs after one month, it is usually attributed to pyrazinamide. Whether toxicity is due to their additive effect, synergistic effect, hypersensitivity phenomenon or direct effect is still not known. Joint Tuberculosis Committee, of British Thoracic Society recommends that liver functions should be monitored weekly in first two weeks, and then at two weekly interval, in patients who have pre-existing liver disease. Recommendation for frequency of monitoring liver functions, in patients with no known risk factors is not clear.

If a patient on antitubercular therapy, develops mild transient elevation of serum bilirubin or liver enzymes, treatment need not to be stopped as they usually come down on continuation of treatment. If patient develops hepatitis related symptoms with significant elevation of bilirubin and liver enzymes, treatment should be stopped and viral hepatitis should be ruled out by serology. Drugs should be gradually reintroduced one by one starting from less hepatotoxic drug first, after liver functions come down to normal, with close monitoring for deterioration.

Antituberculosis Treatment with Pre-existing Liver Disease

In case of stable liver disease, all antitubercular drug could be used, but under close observation for liver functions. In patients with unstable or advanced liver disease, liver function tests should be done at the start of treatment, if possible. If the serum SGPT level is more than 3 times normal before the initiation of treatment, lesser hepatotoxic regimens should be considered. The alternate regimens are devised on the premise that more unstable or severe the liver disease is, fewer the hepatotoxic drugs employed. Possible regimens include those that employ two hepatotoxic drugs (rather than the three in the standard regimen): (a) where 9 months of isoniazid and rifampicin, plus ethambutol (until or unless isoniazid susceptibility is documented) is advocated; or (b) where 2 months of isoniazid, rifampicin, streptomycin and ethambutol is followed by 6–7 months of isoniazid and rifampicin; or (c) where 6–9 months of rifampicin, pyrazinamide and ethambutol is administered.

When the liver disease is too serious to permit use of more than one hepatotoxic drug, then a regimen comprising two months of isoniazid, ethambutol and streptomycin, followed by 10 months of isoniazid and ethambutol is preferred. In the extreme case of fulminant hepatic failure where antitubercular treatment is indispensable, a regimen devoid of any hepatotoxic drug is prescribed; which is 18–24 months of streptomycin, ethambutol and a fluoroquinolone. No dosage adjustment is required in patients with mild to moderate hepatic impairment with bedaquiline and delamanid. Dosing and toxicity not well established in severe hepatic impairment, use with caution and only when the benefits outweigh the risks.

FURTHER READINGS

1. American Thoracic Society/Centers for Disease Control and Prevention/Infectious Diseases Society of America: Treatment of Tuberculosis. Am J Respir Crit Care Med. 2003;167:603-62.
2. Briggs GG, Freeman RK, Yaffe SJ (Eds). Drugs in pregnancy and lactation, 5th edition. Baltimore, MD: Williams & Wilkins. 1998;11:112-7.
3. Chemotherapy and management of tuberculosis in the United Kingdom: recommendations 1998. Thorax. 1998;53:536-648.
4. Companion handbook to the WHO guidelines for the programmatic management of drug-resistant tuberculosis.WHO Geneva; 2014.
5. DOTS PLUS guidelines, Revised National Tuberculosis Control Programme, Central TB Divison Directorate General Health Services, Ministry of Health & Family welfare, Nirman Bhawan, New Delhi. Sep 2008;/Revised National Tuberculosis Control Programme. Guidelines on Programmatic Management of Drug Resistant TB (PMDT) in India. Central TB Division, Directorate General of Health Services, Ministry of Health & Family Welfare, Nirman Bhavan, New Delhi. May 2012.
6. Franks AL, Binkin NJ, Sinder DE Jr, Rokaw WM, Becker S. Isoniazid hepatitis among pregnant and post partum Hispanic patients. Public Health Rep. 1989;104:151-5.
7. Frieden T, Espinal M. What is the therapeutic effect and what is the toxicity of antituberculosis drugs? Toman's Tuberculosis. Case Detection, Treatment and Monitoring, 2nd edition. World Health Organization, Geneva. 2004;110-121.
8. Guidelines for the programmatic management of drug resistant tuberculosis. Emergency Update. 2008;9:82-3.
9. Harries A. How does treatment of tuberculosis differ in patients with pregnancy, liver disease, or renal disease? Toman's Tuberculosis. Case Detection, Treatment and Monitoring, 2nd edition. World Health Organization, Geneva. 2004;166-8.
10. Held H, Fried F. Elimination of para-aminosalicylic acid in patients with renal insufficiency. Chemotherapy. 1977;23:405-15.
11. Malone RS, Fish DN, Spiegel DM, Childs JM, Peloquin CA. The effect of hemodialysis on isoniazid, rifampicin, pyrazinamide and ethambutol. Am J Respir Crit Care Med. 1999;159:1580-4.
12. Nahid P, et al. ATS/CDC/IDSA Clinical Practice Guidelines: Treatment of Drug-Susceptible Tuberculosis. Clin Infec Dis. 2016:1-50.
13. Pande JN, Singh SPN, Khilnani GC, Khilnani S, Tandon R. Risk factors for hepatoxicity from anti tuberculosis drugs: a case control study. Thorax. 1996;51:132-6.
14. Prasad R, Verma SK, Chaudhary SR, Chandra M. Predisposing factors in hepatitis induced by antitubercular regimen containing isoniazid, rifampicin and pyrazinamide: a case control study. Journal of Internal Medicine of India. 2006;9:73-78.
15. Strauss I, Erhardt F. Ethambutol absorption, excretion and dosage in patients with renal tuberculosis. Chemotherapy. 1970;15:148-157.
16. Treatment of Tuberculosis. Guidelines for National Programmes. World Health Organisation document. 2003;annex 2:15-6.
17. WHO Treatment of tuberculosis Guidelines, 4th edition. 2009;8:97-98.

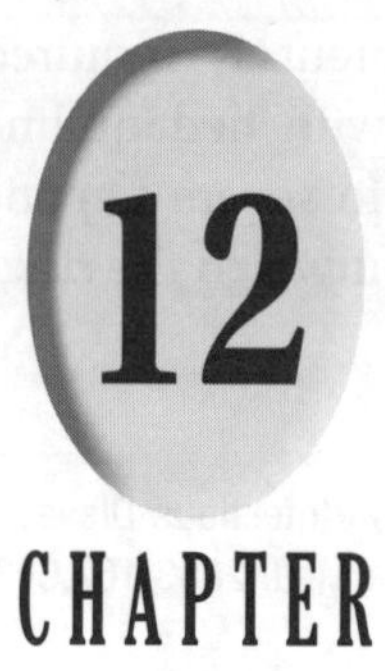

CHAPTER

Treatment of Tuberculosis in Pregnancy, Renal Insufficiency and Liver Diseases: Case-based Approach

TREATMENT OF TB IN PREGNANCY AND LACTATION

Case 1

A 24-year-old, lady having pregnancy of three months, presented with newly diagnosed sputum positive pulmonary tuberculosis. Her liver and renal function were within normal limits. Rifampicin, isoniazid and ethambutol are safe for use in pregnancy. Pyrazinamide is not confidentlyrecommended, because of lack of evidence for safety. Since she was sputum positive, and rapid sputum conversion was needed, she could be given 4 drug regimen of rifampicin, isoniazid, ethambutol and pyrazinamide for 2 months followed by rifampicin and isoniazid for next 4 months, as per World Health Organization (WHO) and International Union Against Tuberculosis and Lung Disease (IUATLD) recommendation, along with prophylactic pyridoxine. The neonate should receive vitamin K injection, to avoid postnatal hemorrhage.

Case 2

A 24-year-old woman having pregnancy of four months, presented with tubercular cervical lymphadenopathy, proved by fine-needle aspiration cytology (FNAC). She also underwent chest skiagram, for any pulmonary lesions, with due precautions for radiation exposure to her fetus. Her liver and renal functions were within normal limits. Since this lady, was suffering from paucibacillary tubercular condition, pyrazinamide may be avoided. This lady may be kept on regimen of rifampicin, isoniazid and ethambutol for 9 months, along with prophylactic pyridoxine.

Case 3

A 26-year-old lady was suffering from, sputum positive pulmonary tuberculosis. She was receiving four drug antitubercular regimen consisting of rifampicin, isoniazid, ethambutol and pyrazinamide, for last one month. While she was on this regimen, she conceived. Since this lady, was already on effective antitubercular drug regimen, there was very little risk of disease to fetus. Drugs being used are considered safe in pregnancy, with some doubt about safety of pyrazinamide. Since she has already taken one month of intensive phase of therapy, she may continue to take same drugs for next one month, following which ethambutol and pyrazinamide may be stopped, and rest of drugs to be continued for next four months.

TREATMENT OF TB IN RENAL INSUFFICIENCY

Case 1

A 33-year-old male weighing 50 kg, presented with sputum positive new case of pulmonary tuberculosis. His liver functions were within normal limits. His renal functions were deranged with value of blood urea as 98 mg/dL and SL creatinine as 4 mg/dL. His creatinine clearance was 18.6 mL/min as calculated by formula as:

Creatinine clearance = {(140 – Age) × Weight in kg}/ 72 × Serum creatinine
(For females above calculated value is multiplied by 0.85)

He may safely be kept on rifampicin and isoniazid without any modificationin dose, or interval of administration. Creatinine clearance level below 30 mL/min raises risk of accumulation of pyrazinoic acid and 5-hydroxyl pyrazinoic acid, which are metabolites of pyrazinamide. Thus, it should be given in dose of 1250 mg (25–35 mg/kg body weight) as three times a week. Streptomycin and ethambutol should preferably be avoided.

Case 2

A 50-year-old female weighing 45 kg, presented with sputum positive pulmonary tuberculosis. She has previously taken antitubercular drugs irregularly for 4 months. Her liver functions were within normal limits. Her renal function was deranged, with blood urea as 84 mg/dL and SL creatinine as 2.25 mg/dL with creatinine clearance of 25 mL/min. This lady should be kept on 5 drug retreatment regimen. Rifampicin and isoniazid are safe in usual doses. Pyrazinamide dose should be altered to 1250 mg three times a week (25–35 mg/kg body weight). Ethambutol and streptomycin, which should preferably be avoided in cases of renal insufficiency, need to be given in this case, but their dose should be modified. Ethambutol could be given in dose of 800 mg three times a week (15–20 mg/kg body weight), streptomycin dose should also be changed to 500 mg three times a week (12–15 mg/kg body weight). If this lady undergoes hemodialysis for management of renal insufficiency, drugs should be given after hemodialysis. Ideally serum concentration of drugs should be regularly monitored, to prevent toxicity, and to ensure therapeutic drug concentration.

Case 3

A 50-year-old man weighing 50 kg, presented with sputum positive pulmonary tuberculosis. He has previously taken irregular treatment, for last three years. His sputum culture on BACTEC was positive for *Mycobacterium tuberculosis*, and bacilli were found resistant to rifampicin and isoniazid. His liver function were within normal limits. His renal functions were deranged with value of blood urea as 74 mg/dL and serum creatinine as 1.05 mg/dL. His creatinine clearance was 60 mL/min. He could have been kept on reserve line drugs. Since renal functions are not very much compromised, he may be given ethionamide, cycloserine and fluoroquinolone. Injectable drugs (e.g. kanamycin) may be given in dose of 500 mg thrice a week (12–15 mg/kg body weight). Para-aminosalicylic acid (PAS) could be used at dose of 4 g twice a day with hemodialysis. Duration of treatment should be 18 to 24 months. Whatever drugs are given, patient should be regularly monitored for serum drug concentration, and renal function, so as to plan and change the medication as and when needed. If this man undergoes hemodialysis, the drugs should be given after it.

Case 4

A 36-year-man weighing 58 kg, presented with sputum positive pulmonary tuberculosis. He has previously taken irregular antitubercular treatment. His sputum culture by BACTEC method was positive for *Mycobacterium tuberculosis*, resistant to rifampicin and isoniazid. His liver functions were within normal limits, but his renal function was impaired with blood urea as 88 mg/dL and serum creatinine as 3.8 mg/dL. His creatinine clearance was 22 mL/min. He should be kept on reserve second line drugs. Severity of renal insufficiency has left us with very little options, which too are risky. Cycloserine should only be used if this patient undergoes hemodialysis, in dose of 500 mg three times a week. Dose of ethionamide should be changed to 250 mg daily (250–500 mg/day). Flouroquinolone dose should also be changed to 750 mg three times a week. Dose of injectable drugs should also be changed to 500 mg three times a week (12–15 mg/kg body weight). PAS is to be avoided. Thioacetazone should not be used.

TREATMENT OF TB IN LIVER DISEASE

Case 1

A 42-year-man presented with fever, anorexia, cough and expectoration for one month. He was diagnosed as a new case of sputum positive pulmonary tuberculosis, and was kept on four drug regimen of rifampicin, isoniazid, ethambutol and pyrazinamide. After 3 weeks he started having vomiting, abdominal pain and yellowish discoloration of eyes and urine. His serum bilirubin was 4.4 mg% and SGPT was 272 IU/L. All of his antitubercular drugs should be stopped, and he should be investigated for viral hepatitis. He should be kept on interim regimen considered safe in liver disease, which should include streptomycin, ethambutol and fluoroquinolone (other than ciprofloxacin). Isoniazid is usually tolerated and can be added in author's opinion. Liver function should be closely monitored. Hepatotoxic drugs like rifampicin and pyrazinamide may be tried one by one after liver function comes down to normal, during frequent monitoring. Many of such patients subsequently tolerate them.

Case 2

A 34-year-woman, with viral hepatitis having HBsAg positive, presented with sputum positive new case of pulmonary tuberculosis. Her renal function were within normal limits. Her serum bilirubin was 7.2 mg% and SGPT was 370 IU/L. Since, this lady is suffering from chronic active liver disease, all hepatotoxic drugs should be avoided. She may be kept on regimen of streptomycin, ethambutol, and fluoroquinolone along with an oral second line drug, preferably cycloserine for 18–24 months. In case her liver function improves on repeat test, in author's experience isoniazid can also be added.

Case 3

A 38-year-man, alcoholic, and a known case of cirrhosis of liver, weighing 48 kg, presented as a case of sputum positive pulmonary tuberculosis. He has taken irregular antitubercular treatment for 3 years, but without response. Current liver function profile showed serum bilirubin as 2.2 mg/dL, SGPT as 312 IU/L, and SGOT as 280 IU/L. His sputum culture on BACTEC was positive for *Mycobacterium tuberculosis*, resistant to isoniazid and rifampicin. He should be given reserve antitubercular drugs. Kanamycin, PAS and fluoroquinolones except ciprofloxacin are safe. Ethionamide could be cautiously used, because of risk of drug-induced hepatotoxicity. Isoniazid may be given in author's opinion, along with supplemental pyridoxine. Cycloserine should not be used, because it can lead to seizures, especially in this case of alcohol related hepatitis. Thioacetazone being hepatotoxic should be avoided. Thus regimen consists of kanamycin, isoniazid, PAS, ethionamide and ofloxacin (K H PAS Ethio Oflo). Duration of treatment should be 18–24 months. Liver function profile should be monitored frequently. Frequency should be weekly for 2 weeks, and then at 2 weekly interval.

FURTHER READINGS

1. Briggs GG, Freeman RK, Yaffe SJ (Eds). Drugs in pregnancy and lactation, 5th edition. Baltimore, MD: Williams & Wilkins. 1998;11:112-7.
2. Chemotherapy and management of tuberculosis in the United Kingdom: recommendations 1998. Thorax. 1998;53:536-648.

3. Companion handbook to the WHO guidelines for the programmatic management of drug-resistant tuberculosis.WHO Geneva; 2014.
4. DOTS PLUS guidelines, Revised National Tuberculosis Control Programme, Central TB Divison Directorate General Health Services, Ministry of Health & Family welfare, Nirman Bhawan, New Delhi. Sep 2008;/Revised National Tuberculosis Control Programme. Guidelines on Programmatic Management of Drug Resistant TB (PMDT) in India. Central TB Division, Directorate General of Health Services, Ministry of Health & Family Welfare, Nirman Bhavan, New Delhi. May 2012.
5. Franks AL, Binkin NJ, Sinder DE Jr, Rokaw WM, Becker S. Isoniazid hepatitis among pregnant and post partum hispanic patients. Public Health Rep. 1989;104:151-5.
6. Frieden T, Espinal M. What is the therapeutic effect and what is the toxicity of antituberculosis drugs? Toman's tuberculosis. Case detection, treatment and monitoring, 2nd edition. World Health Organization, Geneva. 2004;110-21.
7. Guidelines for the programmatic management of drug resistant tuberculosis. Emergency Update. 2008;9:82-3.
8. Harries A. How does treatment of tuberculosis differ in patients with pregnancy, liver disease, or renal disease? Toman's Tuberculosis: Case Detection, Treatment and Monitoring, 2nd edition. World Health Organization, Geneva. 2004;166-8.
9. Held H, Fried F. Elimination of para-aminosalicylic acid in patients with renal insufficiency. Chemotherapy. 1977;23:405-15.
10. Malone RS, Fish DN, Spiegel DM, Childs JM, Peloquin CA. The effect of hemodialysis on isoniazid, rifampicin, pyrazinamide and ethambutol. Am J Respir Crit Care Med. 1999;159:1580-4.
11. Nahid P, et al. ATS/CDC/IDSA Clinical Practice Guidelines: Treatment of Drug-Susceptible Tuberculosis. Clin Infec Dis. 2016:1-50.
12. Pande JN, Singh SPN, Khilnani GC, Khilnani S, Tandon R. Risk factors for hepatoxicity from anti tuberculosis drugs: a case control study. Thorax. 1996;51:132-6.
13. Prasad R, Verma SK, Chaudhary SR, Chandra M. Predisposing factors in Hepatitis induced by antitubercular regimen containing isoniazid, rifampicin and pyrazinamide: A case control study. Journal of Internal Medicine of India. 2006;9:73-8.
14. Strauss I, Erhardt F. Ethambutol absorption, excretion and dosage in patients with renal tuberculosis. Chemotherapy. 1970;15:148-57.
15. WHO Treatment of Tuberculosis Guidelines, 4th edition. 2009;8:97-8.

CHAPTER

Multidrug Resistant Tuberculosis/Rifampicin Resistant Tuberculosis: Principles of Management

Multidrug resistant tuberculosis (MDR-TB) is defined as disease due to *Mycobacterium tuberculosis* that is resistant to isoniazid (H) and rifampicin (R) with or without resistance to other drugs. Rifampicin resistant TB (RR-TB) defined as resistance to rifampicin detected using genotypic or phenotypic methods with or without resistance to other first line anti-TB drugs. MDR-TB/RR-TB has been an area of growing concern to human health worldwide and posing a threat to the control of tuberculosis. The Global Tuberculosis Report 2016 estimated that of 3.9% newly diagnosed and 21% of previously treated Tuberculosis cases had MDR-TB. It has been estimated that 580,000 cases of TB resistant to atleast rifampicin (RR-TB) globally in 2015 of whom 480,000 were having resistant to both rifampicin and isoniazid (MDR-TB) and 250,000 death occurred due to MDR-TB/RR-TB in 2015 globally. In India, estimates showed that the prevalence of MDR-TB among new and previously treated patients was 2.5% and 16% respectively. MDR-TB/RR-TB is emerging as major problem due to poor management of drug sensitive as well as drug resistance TB. MDR-TB/RR-TB is treatable but is very expensive, requires long duration of treatment and contains potentially toxic drugs and treatment success rate is 50–60% only. This write-up aims to discuss the principles of diagnosis and treatment of MDR-TB/RR-TB.

PRINCIPLES OF DIAGNOSIS OF MDR-TB/ RR-TB

Early suspicion, diagnosis and appropriate treatment of MDR–TB/RR-TB is essential to prevent morbidity, mortality and transmission of MDR–TB/RR-TB. An 'presumptive case of MDR-TB ' is defined as a TB patient who fails new treatment regimen and retreatment regimens with first-line anti-TB drugs who is sputum smear positive at the end of the fourth month of treatment or later and close contacts of drug-resistant TB cases. Diagnosis of MDR - TB/RR-TB is based on clinical, radiological and bacteriological evidences. Clinical evidence comprises of the symptoms and signs suggestive of TB and past history of anti-tubercular treatment. History of prior treatment with antitubercular drugs is most important. The main predictor of resistance to a particular drug is the demonstration of its prior use in monotherapy for more than one month. To obtain evidence of possible inadvertent or direct monotherapy, it is essential to be meticulous in obtaining the history of anti-tuberculosis treatment in all presumptive cases of MDR-TB. There should be a detailed evaluation into the drugs used, the drug dosages if previous drug prescriptions are available, whether the drugs were fixed dose combinations or separate drugs, their reliability in terms of WHO approved bioavailability, whether the patients were compliant to these drugs, supervised or unsupervised treatment and any drug intolerance that included partial or complete drug defaulting. Any real masked monotherapy previously received by the patient can be identified with reasonably good accuracy and one can accurately predict resistance to specific drugs and prevent their inclusion in the retreatment plan. The other important aspects of history include contacts with known case of resistant tuberculosis and patient's place of residence which may have a high prevalence of drug resistance. Though radiological worsening is not a very reliable indicator for predicting drug resistance, it serves to compliment the clinical and bacteriological evidence of the patient. Change in size of cavities and increase in size of existing lesions and appearance of new lesions are signs of disease progression and activity.

The bacteriological evidence serve as the gold standard in the detection of MDR -TB/RR-TB. This is based on sputum smear microscopy and culture of *M. tuberculosis* and drug susceptibility testing (DST). Sputum smear microscopy, after starting standard chemotherapy can show a positive, negative or suboptimal response. While positive response is characterized by sputum conversion at 2/3 months of chemotherapy, a negative response could mean persistent smear positivity at the end of 3 months of adequate chemotherapy and a suboptimal response by an initial fall in the sputum grade followed by a gradual rise—the so called 'fall and rise' phenomenon while the patient is on antitubercular treatment. The last two patterns increase the probability of drug resistant tuberculosis. Diagnosis is confirmed by DST from reliable and reputed laboratories under constant quality control. However, one has to keep in mind the limitation of highly specific DST because the technique is complex, difficult to perform accurately even when skilled personnel are available and laboratory facilities are of high standard. Further one should realize that laboratories vary in reliability; errors may occur in laboratories, different DST reports are obtained from the same patient from different laboratories. There is often lack of standardization, coordination and cross checking by national and supranational reference laboratories. Susceptibility testing for isoniazid, rifampicin, flouroquinolones and the injectables drugs (kanamycin, amikacin, capreomycin) is very reliable. For other drugs it is less reliable and basing individualized treatments on DST for these drugs should be avoided. The effectiveness or ineffectiveness of a drug cannot be predicted by DST with 100% certainty. Furthermore, the DST to second line drugs (SLD'S) is very variable. Keeping above facts in mind it is pertinent that DST should not be accepted uncritically.

Molecular techniques have been used for identification of resistance associated mutation. WHO with stop TB partnership endorsed line probe assays (LPA) in low resource countries in 2008. LPA's can do rapid screening of patients with MDR-TB/RR-TB risk within 2 days. The Xpert MTB RIF assay endorsed by WHO in 2010 enables simultaneous detection of *M. tuberculosis* and rifampicin resistance (reliable proxy for MDR-TB) directly from sputum and other extrapulmonary specimen except blood in less than 2 hours. The assay is robust enough to be performed outside of conventional laboratories at district and sub-district level of health system but requires uninterrupted power supply. It provides accurate results and can allow rapid initiation of MDR-TB/RR-TB treatment pending results from conventional culture and DST. WHO recently recommended 2nd line probe assay (2nd LPA), a rapid diagnostic test MTBDRsL that identifies genetic mutation in MDR strains that detect resistance to flouroquinolones and injectable second line anti-TB drugs.

PRINCIPLES OF TREATMENT OF MDR-TB/ RR-TB

For treatment of MDR-TB/RR-TB, standardized, empirical and individualized approaches have been laid down. Individualized treatment based on individual DST and prior treatment history is costly and needs skilled professionals, standardized treatment is simple, less costly and same treatment is given to all patients. Designing an individualized appropriate regimen need skill and treatment of MDR-TB/RR-TB is very difficult in the hands of many physicians with restricted knowledge who dare to treat these patients and create worsening problems. Therefore individualized treatment needs specialized physicians experienced in dealing with such cases since this treatment represents the patient's last chance of a cure.

Ideally, an appropriate treatment regimen should consist of pyrazinamide and atleast 4 new drugs selected from 5 groups of anti-TB drugs in hierarchical order which the patient has not taken previously or to which bacilli is considered to be sensitive but WHO has reclassified the anti-TB drugs used for MDR-TB in 2016 in 4 groups—A, B, C and D. In patients with MDR-TB/RR-TB, a regimen with at least five effective anti-TB drugs during the intensive phase is recommended, including pyrazinamide and four core second-line Anti-TB drugs—one chosen from group A (flouroquinolones: levofloxacin, moxifloxacin and gatifloxacin), one from group B (second line injectable drugs: kanamycin, amikacin, capreomycin), and at least two from group C (Other core second-line drugs: ethionamide/prothionamide, cycloserine/terizidone, linezolid and clofazimine). If the minimum of effective anti-TB cannot be composed as above, one drug from group D2 (bedaquiline and delamanid) and other drugs from D3 (PAS, Imipenem-cilastatin, meropenem, amoxicillin-clavulanate and thioacetazone) may be added to bring the total no. of drugs to five. The regimen may be further strengthened with rest of Group D1 (high-dose isoniazid and/or ethambutol). While streptomycin is not usually included with the second-line drugs it can be used as the injectable drug of the core MDR-TB regimen if none of the three other injectable drugs can be used and if the strain can be reliably shown not to be resistant. Thioacetazone should not be used if the patient is HIV seropositive. Intensive phase including injectables should be given for atleast 8 months for most patients which can be modified depending upon the response of the patient and the total duration of treatment is atleast 20 months which can be prolonged up to 24 months depending upon the response of the patient. Pyrazinamide is usually continued for the entire treatment especially if there is extensive disease. If the patient has minimal disease, pyrazinamide can be stopped with injectables at end of intensive phase. Bedaquiline or delamanid are used for 6 months in intensive phase and are presently not recommended for whole treatment duration.

A new shorter regimen for treatment for subset of MDR-TB/RR-TB patients have been introduced recently. In patients with MDR-TB/RR-TB who have not been previously treated with second-line drugs and in whom resistance to flouroquinolones and second-line injectable agents has been excluded or is considered highly unlikely, a shorter MDR-TB regimen of 9–12 months may be used instead of a conventional regimen of 20–24 months. The intensive phase of 4 months which may be extended to 6 months in case of lack of sputum smear conversion consists of gatifloxacin or moxifloxacin, kanamycin, prothionamide, clofazimine, high-dose isoniazid, pyrazinamide, and ethambutol. This is followed by a continuation phase of 5 months which consist of gatifloxacin or moxifloxacin, clofazimine, ethambutol, and pyrazinamide.

Extrapulmonary MDR-TB/RR-TB is treated with the same regimen and duration as pulmonary MDR-TB/RR-TB. If the patient has symptoms suggestive of central nervous system involvement and is infected with MDR-TB/RR-TB, the regimen should use drugs that have adequate penetration into the central nervous system. Rifampicin, isoniazid, pyrazinamide, prothionamide/ethionamide and cycloserine have good penetration into the cerebrospinal fluid (CSF); kanamycin, amikacin and capreomycin do so only in the presence of meningeal inflammation; PAS and ethambutol have poor or no penetration. The flouroquinolones have variable CSF penetration, with better penetration seen in the later generations. Linezolid is believed to penetrate the central nervous system, and has been used in meningitis treatment. Imipenem has good central nervous system penetration, but children with meningitis treated with imipenem had high rates of seizures and meropenem is preferred for meningitis cases and children· There is no data on central nervous system penetration of clofazimine, clarithromycin, bedaquiline and delamanid.

It is important that a single drug should never be added to a failing regimen and it is ineffective to combine 2 drugs of the same group or to add a drug potentially ineffective because of cross resistance. No drug should be kept in reserve and the most powerful drugs should be used initially and in maximum combination so as to ensure that first battle is won and won permanently. All patients initiated on treatment and their family members should be intensively counseled prior to treatment initiation and during all follow up visits. To reduce the risk of development of resistance to second line anti-TB drugs and promote optimal treatment outcomes, all efforts should be made to administer treatment under direct observation (DOT) over the entire course of treatment. If DOT is not possible, attempts to ensure treatment adherence should be made by checking empty blister packs during follow-up visits every month. All measures should be taken to persuade and encourage patients not to stop treatment despite all its discomforts as it is the last resort that stands between life and death. Surgical treatment should be considered as an adjunct to chemotherapy whenever applicable and when results of chemotherapy are very unpredictable.

Adjuvant use of corticosteroids can be beneficial in conditions like severe central nervous system or pericardial involvement. Corticosteroids do not increase mortality when the patient is on effective regimen and should be used with tapering of doses over several weeks. The immunomodulators may have the potential to improve outcomes in all TB including MDR-TB/RR-TB as seen in evidence reviewed by expert group in 2007 but still evaluation of efficacy and safety of such therapy is needed before any recommendation is made.

MDR-TB/RR-TB treatment should include nutritional assessment and counseling of the all patients. Because of disease process patient appetite is reduced and tends to be malnourished, in addition, second line anti-TB drugs can further reduce appetite. Patients should be properly counseled for adequate food intake. One such step is to provide free food which is thought to improve quality of life and may improve treatment adherence but further research is necessary. Addition of vitamins probably does not improve weight gain and also no studies have assessed their effect on quality of life but they may be added to treat specific deficiencies like vitamin A. Furthermore, vitamin B_6 should be given if treatment regimen consists of cycloserine, terizidone, high dose isoniazid or linezolid to prevent neurological side effects.

CONCLUSION

Treatment of MDR-TB/RR-TB is difficult, complicated, much costlier, challenging and needs experience and skills. MDR-TB/RR-TB is a human made problem and its emergence can be prevented by prompt diagnosis and effective treatment of all TB case. Adoption of directly observed treatment short course (DOTS) to prevent the MDR-TB/RR-TB and careful introduction of second line drugs to treat patients with MDR-TB/RR-TB are the top priorities for the proper management of MDR-TB/RR-TB and to prevent development of extensively drug resistant tuberculosis (XDR-TB).

FURTHER READINGS

1. Caminero JA. Management of multidrug-resistant tuberculosis and patients in retreatment. Eur Respir J. 2005;25:928-36.
2. Companion Handbook to the WHO guidelines for the programmatic management of drug resistant tuberculosis. WHO/HTM/TB/2014.11
3. Dom´inguez J, Boettger EC, Cirillo D, Cobelens F, Eisenach KD, Gagneux S, et al. Clinical implications of molecular drug resistance testing for *Mycobacterium tuberculosis*: a TBNET/ *RESIST-TB consensus Statement*. Int J Tuberc Lung Dis. 2016; 20: 24-42.
4. Guidelines for programmatic management of drug resistant tuberculosis. WHO, 2011. WHO/ HTM/TB/2011.6.
5. Holdiness MR. Cerebrospinal fluid pharmokinetics of antituberculosis drugs. Clinical Pharmacokinetics. 1985; 10:532-4.
6. International Union Against Tuberculosis and Lung Diseases. Guidelines for Clinical and Operational Management of Drug-Resistant Tuberculosis. IUTLD. Paris; 2013.
7. Kim SJ. Drug susceptibility testing in tuberculosis: methods and reliability of results. E Respir J. 2005; 25:564-9.
8. Lund DI, Zwerling AA, Pai M. Genotype MTB DR assays for the diagnosis of multi drug resistant tuberculosis: a meta-analysis. ERJ. 2008;32;1165-74.
9. Management of patients with multidrug resistant/extensively drug-resistant tuberculosis in Europe: a TBNET consensus statement. ERJ. 2014; 44:23-63.
10. Prasad R, Singh A, Srivastava R, Kushwaha RAS, Garg R , Verma SK; et al. Treatment outcome of multi drug resistant tuberculosis patients in modified DOTS PLUS. ERJ. 2012; 40: (suppl 56) p. 3321(abstract).
11. Prasad R, Verma SK, Sahai S, Kumar S, Jain A. Efficacy and safety of kanamycin, ethionamide, PAS and cycloserine in multidrug resistant pulmonary tuberculosis patients. Indian J Chest Dis Allied Sci. 2006; 48:181-4.
12. Report of the expert consultation on immunotherapeutic interventions for tuberculosis. Geneva: World Health Organization, 2007.
13. Steingart KR, Schiller I, Horne DJ, Pai M, Boehme CC, Dendukuri N. Xpert MTB/RIF assay for pulmonary tuberculosis and rifampicin resistance in adults. Cochrane database Syst Rev. 2014 Jan 21;1:Cd009593.
14. The use of molecular line probe assays for the detection of resistance to second-line anti-tuberculosis drugs. WHO/HTM/TB/2016.07.
15. Treatment of Tuberculosis: Guidelines, 4th edition. WHO\HTM\TB\2009.420.
16. WHO treatment guidelines for drug-resistant tuberculosis 2016 update. WHO/HTM/ TB/2016.04.

17. World Health Organization. Global Tuberculosis Report 2016. WHO/HTM/2016.13.Geneva World Health Organization; 2016.
18. World Health Organization. Policy statement: automated real-time nucleic acid amplification technology for rapid and simultaneous detection of tuberculosis and rifampicin resistance: Xpert MTB/RIF system. Geneva, World Health Organization; 2011.
19. World Health Organization. Policy update. Xpert MTB/RIF assays fro the diagnosis of pulmonary and extrapulmonary TB in adults and children. WHO/HTM/TB/2013.6. Geneva, Switzerland: WHO; 2013.

CHAPTER

Treatment of Multidrug Resistant and Extensively Drug Resistant Tuberculosis in Special Situations

Compared to drug sensitive tuberculosis, Multidrug Resistant and Extensively Drug Resistant Tuberculosis (M/XDR-TB) is more demanding in terms of cost of treatment, duration of treatment, higher adverse reactions to second-line drugs, resources required by the treatment providers, and the prolonged adherence required by the patients. To add to these issues, certain associated special situations make the treatment of multidrug resistant and extensively drug resistant tuberculosis (M/XDR-TB) more difficult. This current review outlines the management of M/XDR-TB in special situations like pregnancy, breastfeeding, contraception, children, diabetes mellitus, renal insufficiency, liver disorders, seizure disorders, psychiatric disorders and substance dependence.

MANAGEMENT OF M/XDR-TB IN PREGNANCY

There is a lack of experience in treating pregnant women with M/XDR-TB. Although teratogenicity has been demonstrated in only a few of the drugs used to treat M/XDR-TB, all except ethambutol have uncertain safety information available. This all makes treating M/XDR-TB during pregnancy very challenging. It is prudent to solicit the opinion of an experienced gynecologist/obstetrician and chest physician while treating such patients. All female patients of childbearing age should be tested for pregnancy upon initial evaluation. Pregnancy is not a contraindication for treatment of M/XDR-TB, which poses great risks to the lives of both mother and fetus. However, birth control is strongly recommended for all non-pregnant women receiving therapy for M/XDR-TB because of the potential consequences for both mother and fetus resulting from frequent and severe adverse drug reactions. M/XDR-TB patients found to be pregnant prior to treatment initiation or on treatment are evaluated taking into consideration the factors like: risks and benefits of M/XDR-TB treatment, severity of the M/XDR-TB, gestational age and potential risk to the fetus. The risks and benefits of treatment should be carefully considered, with the primary goal of smear conversion to protect the health of the mother and child, both before and after birth. Since the majority of teratogenic effects occur in the first trimester, therapy may be delayed until the second trimester. The decision to postpone the start of treatment should be agreed by both patient and doctor after analysis of the risks and benefits. The decision is based primarily on clinical judgment established on the basis of severity of the disease. When therapy is started, treat with three or four oral second-line anti-TB drugs which are likely to be highly effective against the infecting strain plus pyrazinamide. The regimen should be reinforced with an injectable agent and other drugs as needed immediately postpartum. For the most part, aminoglycosides should not be used in the regimens of pregnant patients and can be particularly toxic to the developing fetal ear. Capreomycin may also carry a risk of ototoxicity but is the injectable drug of choicc if an injectable agent cannot be avoided. The option of using capreomycin thrice weekly from the start can be considered to decrease drug exposure to the fetus. Ethionamide can increase the risk of nausea and vomiting associated with pregnancy, and teratogenic effects have been observed in animal studies. If possible, ethionamide should be avoided in pregnant patients. Consider termination of pregnancy if the mother's life is compromised. When the condition of the mother is so poor that a pregnancy would carry a significant risk to her life, a medical abortion may be indicated. Further management of M/XDR-TB patients who are pregnant prior to initiation of M/XDR-TB treatment or whilst on M/XDR-TB treatment are based on the duration of pregnancy. If the duration of pregnancy is <20 weeks, the patient should be advised to opt for a medical termination of pregnancy (MTP) in view of the potential severe risk to both the mother and fetus. If the patient is willing, she should be referred to a Gynecologist/ Obstetrician for MTP following which M/XDR-TB treatment can be initiated if the patient has not started M/XDR-TB treatment or continued if the patient is already on M/XDR-TB treatment. For patients who are unwilling for MTP or have pregnancy of >20 weeks, the risk to the mother and fetus needs to be explained clearly and a modified treatment for M/XDR-TB should be started. For patients in the first trimester (≤12 weeks), kanamycin and ethionamide are omitted from the M/XDR-TB regimen and PAS is added. For patients who have completed the first trimester (>12 weeks), kanamycin is replaced with PAS. Postpartum, PAS may be replaced with kanamycin and continued until the end of the intensive phase. Pregnant M/XDR-TB patients need to be monitored carefully both in relation to the treatment and the progress of the pregnancy. This approach should lead to good results, since the patient should be smear negative at the time of parturition, and mother and infant do not need to be separated. Breastfeeding should be encouraged as long as the patient is sputum negative.

Despite limited data on safety and long-term use of fluoroquinolones, cycloserine, para-aminosalicylic acid (PAS) and amoxicillin/clavulanate in pregnancy, they are considered the drug of choice for M/XDR-TB treatment during pregnancy. If the injectable agents, ethionamide/prothionamide, or other drugs were withheld because of the pregnancy, they can be added back postpartum to make a more complete regimen. There may not be a clear transition between the intensive phase and continuation phase, and the injectable agent can be given for three to six months postpartum even in the middle of treatment. Alternatively, if the patient is doing well and past the normal eight-month period for the injectable agent, it need not be added. The total treatment duration is the same as for M/XDR-TB treatment. The child should receive Bacillus Calmette–Guérin (BCG) vaccination at birth as per WHO policy. As there is limited data on safety of delamanid and bedaquiline in pregnancy for treatment of M/XDR-TB, these drugs should be avoided.

MANAGEMENT OF M/XDR-TB IN BREASTFEEDING

Timely and properly applied chemotherapy is the best way to prevent transmission of tubercle bacilli to the baby. A woman who is breastfeeding and has drug-resistant TB should receive a full course of antituberculosis treatment. In lactating mothers on treatment, most antituberculosis drugs will be found in the breast milk in concentrations that would equal only a small fraction of the therapeutic dose used in an infant. However, any effect on infants of such exposure during the full course of M/XDR-TB treatment have not been established. Therefore, when resources are available, it is recommended to provide infant formula options as an alternative to breastfeeding. The mother and her baby should not be completely separated. However, if the mother is sputum smear-positive, the care of the infant should be left to family members until she becomes sputum smear-negative, if this is feasible. When the mother and infant are together, this common time should be spent in well-ventilated areas or outdoors. In some settings, the mother may be offered the option of using a surgical mask or an N-95 respirator until she becomes sputum smear-negative.

MANAGEMENT OF M/XDR-TB IN CONTRACEPTION

All women of child-bearing age who are receiving M/XDR-TB therapy should be advised to use birth-control measures because of the potential risk to both mother and fetus. There is no contraindication to the use of oral contraceptives with the non-rifamycin containing regimens. It should be remembered that oral contraceptives might have decreased efficacy due to vomiting and drug interactions with second-line drugs. These patients should be advised to take their contraceptives apart from times when they may experience vomiting caused by the antituberculosis treatment. Patients who vomit at any time directly after, or within the first two hours after, taking the contraceptive tablet, should use a barrier method of contraception until a full month of the contraceptive tablets can be tolerated. Thus for prevention of pregnancy, the use of barrier methods (condoms/diaphragm), intrauterine devices (IUDs) or medroxyprogesterone are recommended based on individual preference and eligibility. Similarly, all women of child bearing age identified as DR-TB suspects should be advised to use a reliable and appropriate contraceptive method till the results of culture and drug susceptibility test (DST) are available. For patients with mono- and poly-resistant TB that is susceptible to rifampicin, the use of rifampicin interacts with the contraceptive drugs resulting in decreased efficacy of protection against pregnancy. A woman on oral contraception while receiving rifampicin treatment may choose between two options: following consultation with a physician, use of an oral contraceptive pill containing a higher dose of estrogen (50 μg); or use of another form of contraception. Condoms are a reasonable solution for patients who do not want to take additional pills and/or when protection against sexually transmitted diseases is also needed. Medroxyprogesterone intramuscular injections and other methods of contraception can also be considered.

MANAGEMENT OF M/XDR-TB IN CHILDREN

There is only limited reported experience with the use of second-line drugs for extended periods in children. Discussion with family members is critical, especially at the outset of therapy. The risks and benefits of each drug should be carefully considered in designing a regimen. Children with drug-resistant TB generally have primary resistance transmitted from an index case with drug resistant TB. When DST is available it should be used to guide therapy, although children with paucibacillary TB are often culture-negative. Nevertheless, every effort should be made to confirm drug-resistant TB bacteriologically by the use of DST and to avoid exposing children unnecessarily to toxic drugs. The treatment of culture-negative children with clinical evidence of active TB disease and contact with a documented case of drug-resistant TB should be guided by the results of DST and the history of the contact's exposure to antituberculosis drugs. M/XDR-TB is a life-threatening condition and no antituberculosis drugs are absolutely contraindicated in children. New anti-TB drugs that have recently been introduced into the market have no safety data on children and should be considered for use in any extreme life-threatening cases, with risk/benefits fully disclosed, and intense safety monitoring. Children who have received treatment for drug-resistant TB have generally tolerated the second-line drugs well. Although fluoroquinolones have been shown to retard cartilage development in beagle puppies, experience in humans has not demonstrated similar effects. It is considered that the benefit of fluoroquinolones in treating M/XDR-TB in children outweighs any risk. Additionally, ethionamide, PAS and cycloserine have been used effectively in children and are well tolerated. In general, dose of antituberculosis drugs should be according to body weight. Monthly monitoring of body weight is therefore especially important in pediatric cases, with adjustment of doses as children gain weight. Dose of all drugs, including the fluoroquinolones, should be given at the higher end of the recommended ranges whenever possible, except ethambutol. Ethambutol should be dosed at 15 mg/kg, and not at 25 mg/kg as sometimes used in adults with M/XDR-TB, as it is more difficult to monitor for optic neuritis in children. In children who are not culture-positive initially, treatment failure is difficult to assess. Persistent abnormalities on chest radiograph do not necessarily signify a lack of improvement. In children, weight loss or, more commonly, failure to gain weight adequately, is of particular concern and often one of the first signs of treatment failure. This is another key reason to monitor weight carefully in children. Anecdotal evidence suggests that adolescents are at high risk for poor treatment outcomes. Early diagnosis, strong social support, individual and family counseling and a close relationship with the medical provider may help to improve outcomes in this group.

MANAGEMENT OF M/XDR-TB IN DIABETES MELLITUS

Diabetes must be managed closely throughout the treatment of M/XDR-TB. The health care provider should be in close communication with the physician who manages the patient's diabetes. Diabetic patients with M/XDR-TB are at risk for poor outcomes. In addition, the presence of diabetes mellitus may potentiate the adverse effects of antitituberculosis drugs, especially renal dysfunction and peripheral neuropathy. Oral hypoglycemic agents are not contraindicated during the treatment of M/XDR-TB but may require the patient to increase the dosage. Use of ethionamide or prothionamide may make it more difficult to control insulin levels. Creatinine and potassium levels should be monitored more frequently, often weekly for the first month and then at least monthly thereafter.

MANAGEMENT OF M/XDR-TB IN RENAL INSUFFICIENCY

Renal insufficiency due to long-standing TB disease itself, previous use of aminoglycosides or concurrent renal disease, is not uncommon. Great care should be taken in the administration of second-line drugs in patients with renal impairment. The dosing is based on the patient's creatinine clearance, which is an estimate of the glomerular filtration rate. Creatinine clearance is calculated by formula Weight (kg) × (140–age) × (constant)/serum creatinine (μmol/L) (constant in the formula is = 1.23 for men and 1.04 for women). Consideration needs to be taken that M/XDR-TB patients require aminoglycosides for 6 months or more. Other drugs, which also might require dose or interval adjustment in presence of mild to moderate renal impairment are ethambutol, quinolones, cycloserine and PAS. In the presence of severe renal impairment many other drugs may also require adjustments as given in Table 14.1. In M/XDR-TB patients, blood urea and serum creatinine should be monitored prior to treatment initiation, monthly for three months after treatment initiation and then every three months whilst injection kanamycin is being administered. In patients with mild renal impairment, the dose of aminoglycosides may be reduced. In the presence of severe renal failure, the aminoglycoside therapy should be discontinued and replaced with other potent non-nephrotoxic antituberculosis drugs.

TABLE 14.1: Dosing recommendation for adult patients with renal insufficiency or undergoing hemodialysis.

Drug	Change in frequency	Dose and frequency in patients with creatinine clearance <30 mL/min or those on hemodialysis
Isoniazid	No change needed	300 mg daily or 900 mg thrice a week
Rifampicin	No change needed	600 mg daily or 600 mg thrice a week
Pyrazinamide	Yes	25–35 mg/kg per dose three times a week
Ethambutol	Yes	15–25 mg/kg per dose three times a week
Rifabutin	No	Normal dose can be used, if possible monitor drug concentrations to avoid toxicity
Rifapentine	No	No adjustment necessary
Levofloxacin	Yes	750–1000 mg per dose three times a week
Moxifloxacin	No	No adjustment necessary
Gatifloxacin	No	400 mg three times a week
Ofloxacin	Yes	600–800 mg per dose three times per week
Cycloserine	Yes	250 mg daily or 500 mg three times a week.
Terizidone		Recommendations not available
Ethionamide	No change needed	250–500 mg daily
PAS	No change needed	4 g/dose twice daily
Streptomycin	Yes	12–15 mg/kg/dose twice or three times a week
Capreomycin	Yes	12–15 mg/kg/dose twice or three times a week
Kanamycin	Yes	12–15 mg/kg/dose twice or three times a week
Amikacin	Yes	12–15 mg/kg/dose twice or three times a week
Clarithromycin	Yes	Usual dose 500 mg twice daily but can be reduced to 250 mg twice daily
Linezolid	No change needed	Usual dose is 600 mg twice daily but can be reduced to 600 mg once daily after 4–6 weeks
Clofazimine	Yes	Begin with 300 mg daily and decreased to 100 mg daily after 4–6 weeks

Contd...

Contd...

Drug	Change in frequency	Dose and frequency in patients with creatinine clearance <30 mL/min or those on hemodialysis
Amoxicillin and clavulanic acid	Yes	Dose used is 625 mg twice daily, 1000 mg should not be used
Bedaquiline	No	No dosage adjustment is required in patients with mild to moderate renal impairment (dosing not established in severe renal impairment, use with caution)
Delamanid	No	No dosage adjustment is required in patients with mild to moderate renal impairment (dosing not established in severe renal impairment, use with caution)
Imipenem/ cilastatin	Yes	For creatinine clearance 20–40 mL/min dose 500 mg every 8 hours; for creatinine clearance <20 mL/min dose 500 mg every 12 hours
Meropenem	Yes	For creatinine clearance 20–40 mL/min dose 750 mg every 12 hours; for creatinine clearance <20 mL/min dose 500 mg every 12 hours
High dose isoniazid		Recommendations not available

MANAGEMENT OF M/XDR-TB IN LIVER DISORDERS

Pyrazinamide is the most hepatotoxic of the three first-line drugs (Rifampicin, isoniazid, pyrazinamide). Rifampicin is least likely to cause hepatocellular damage, although it is associated with cholestatic jaundice. Among the second-line drugs, ethionamide, prothionamide and PAS can also be hepatotoxic, although less so than any of the first-line drugs. Hepatitis occurs rarely with the flouroquinolones. The potential for hepatotoxicity is increased in elderly, alcoholics and in patients with pre-existing liver disease. In general, most of second-line drugs can be safely used in presence of mild hepatic impairment, as they are relatively less hepatotoxic than the first-line drugs. However, pyrazinamide should be avoided in such patients. All other drugs can be used, but close monitoring of liver enzymes is advised. If significant aggravation of liver inflammation occurs, the drugs responsible may have to be stopped. Once a patient on second-line drugs develops hepatitis, other etiologies should also be excluded such as viral hepatitis, alcoholic hepatitis, drug-induced hepatitis by non-TB drugs. Uncommonly, a patient with TB may have concurrent acute hepatitis that is unrelated to TB or anti-TB treatment; and here clinical judgment becomes necessary. In some cases, it is possible to defer anti-TB treatment until the acute hepatitis has been resolved. In other cases when it is necessary to treat drug-resistant TB during acute hepatitis, the combination of four non-hepatotoxic drugs is the safest option. Viral hepatitis should be treated if medically indicated and treatment can occur during drug-resistant TB treatment.

MANAGEMENT OF M/XDR-TB IN SEIZURE DISORDERS

TB might itself involve central nervous system and may cause seizures. However, when seizures are present for the first time during anti-TB therapy, they are likely to be the result of an adverse effect of one of the anti-TB drugs. Among second-line drugs, cycloserine, ethionamide and fluoroquinolones have been associated with seizures. High dose isoniazid also carries a high risk of seizure and should be avoided in patients with active seizure disorders. Some patients requiring treatment for M/XDR-TB will have a past or present medical history of a seizure disorder. The first step in evaluating such patients is to determine whether the seizure disorder is under control and whether the patient is taking anti-seizure medication to control the disorder. If the seizures are not under control, initiation or adjustment of anti-seizure medications will be needed prior to the start of M/XDR-TB therapy. In addition, if other underlying conditions or causes for seizures exist, they should be corrected. Pyridoxine should be given with cycloserine to prevent seizures. The suggested prophylactic dose for at-risk patients on isoniazid is 10 to 25 mg/day and for patients on cycloserine is 25 mg of pyridoxine for every 250 mg of cycloserine daily. Cycloserine should however be avoided in patients with active seizure disorders that are not well controlled with medication. In cases where no other drug is appropriate, cycloserine can be given and the anti-seizure medication adjusted as needed to control the seizure disorder. The risk and benefits of using cycloserine should be discussed with the patient and the decision on whether to use cycloserine are made together with the patient. Antiepileptic drugs like phenytoin increases metabolism of cycloserine and quinolones leading to low serum concentration. Therefore, high dose of cycloserine and quinolones may be required in patients with seizure disorder on antiepileptic medications. Hence, close monitoring of serum levels of antiepileptic drugs should be done preferably, if facility exists.

MANAGEMENT OF M/XDR-TB IN SUBSTANCE DEPENDENCE

Patients with substance dependence disorders should be offered treatment for addiction. Complete abstinence from alcohol or other substances should be strongly encouraged, although active consumption is not a contraindication for antituberculosis treatment. If the treatment is repeatedly interrupted because of the patient's dependence, therapy should be suspended until successful treatment or measures to ensure adherence have been established. Good Directly Observed Therapy (DOT) gives the patient contact with and support from health-care providers, which often allows complete treatment even in patients with substance dependence. Cycloserine will have a higher incidence of adverse effects in patients dependent on alcohol or other substances, including higher incidence of seizures. However, if cycloserine is considered important to the regimen, it should be used and the patient closely observed for adverse effects, which are then adequately treated.

M/XDR-TB IN PATIENTS WITH PSYCHOSIS

There is a high baseline incidence of depression and anxiety in patients with M/XDR-TB, often connected with the chronicity and socioeconomic stress factors related to the disease. For M/XDR-TB patients with a concurrent psychiatric illness, it is advisable to have an evaluation carried out by a psychiatrist before the start of treatment for M/XDR-TB. The initial evaluation documents any pre-existing psychiatric condition and establishes a baseline for comparison if new psychiatric symptoms develop while the patient is on treatment. Any identified psychiatric illness at the start or during treatment should be fully addressed. If a health care worker with psychiatric training is not available, the treating health care provider should document any psychiatric conditions the patient may have at the initial evaluation. Treatment with psychiatric medication, individual counseling, and/or group therapy may be necessary to manage the patient suffering from a psychiatric condition or adverse psychiatric effect due to medication. Fluoroquinolones and ethionomide have been associated with psychosis. Pyridoxine prophylaxis may minimize risk of neurologic and psychiatric adverse reactions. Cycloserine may cause severe psychosis and depression leading to suicidal tendencies. However the use of cycloserine is not absolutely contraindicated for the psychiatric patient. Adverse effects of cycloserine may be more prevalent in the psychiatric patient, but the benefits of using this drug often outweigh the potential higher risk of adverse effects. Close monitoring is recommended if cycloserine is used in patients with psychiatric disorders. If patient on cycloserine therapy develops psychosis, antipsychotic treatment should be started and cycloserine therapy should be temporarily suspended. Once symptoms resolve and patient is stabilized, cycloserine therapy may be resumed. Such patients may require antipsychotic treatment till anti-TB treatment is completed. When any patient on M/XDR-TB treatment develops psychosis, other etiologies such as psychosocial stresses, depression, hypothyroidism, illicit drug and alcohol use, should also be looked for.

FURTHER READINGS

1. Brost BC, Newman RB. The maternal and fetal effects of tuberculosis therapy. Obstetrics and Gynecology Clinics of North America. 1997;24:659-73.
2. Companion Handbook to the WHO guidelines for the programmatic management of drug resistant tuberculosis. WHO/HTM/TB/2014.11.

3. Drobac PC, del Castillo H, Sweetland A, Anca G, Joseph JK, Furin J, Shin S. Treatment of multidrug-resistant tuberculosis during pregnancy: long-term follow-up of 6 children with intrauterine exposure to second-line agents. Clin Infect Dis. 2005;40:1689-92.
4. Duff P. Antibiotic selection in obstetric patients. Infect Dis Clin North Am. 1997;11:1-12.
5. Figueroa-Damian R, Arredondo-Garcia JL. Neonatal outcome of children born to women with tuberculosis. Archives of Medical Research. 2001;32:66-9.
6. Guidelines for programmatic management of drug resistant tuberculosis. WHO, 2011. WHO/HTM/TB/2011.6
7. Guidelines for the programmatic management of drug-resistant tuberculosis: emergency update 2008. Geneva, World Health Organization, 2008 (WHO/HTM/TB/ 2008.402).
8. Hamadeh MA, Glassroth J. Tuberculosis and Pregnancy: Chest. 1992;101:1114-20.1.
9. Hampel B, Hullmann R, Schmidt H. Ciprofloxacin in pediatrics: worldwide clinical experience based on compassionate use–safety report. Pediatric Infectious Disease Journal. 1997;16:127-29.
10. Lansdown FS, Beran M, Litwak T. Psychotoxic reaction during ethionamide therapy. Am Rev Resp Dis. 1967;95:1053-5.
11. Loebstein R, Koren G. Clinical pharmacology and therapeutic drug monitoring in neonates and children. Pediatric Review. 1998;19:422-8.
12. Mukherjee JS, Joseph JK, Rich ML, Shin SS, Furin JJ, Seung KJ, et al. Clinical and programmatic considerations in the treatment of MDR-TB in children: a series of 16 patients from Lima, Peru. Int J Tuber Lung Dis. 2003;7:637-44.
13. Patel AM, McKeon J. Avoidance and management of adverse reactions to antituberculosis drugs. Drugs. 1995;12:1-25.
14. Prasad R, Gupta N. MDR and XDR Tuberculosis. Jaypee Brothers Medical Publishers, 1st edition. 2015, pp. 112-19.
15. Ruckenstein MI. Vertigo and disequilibrium with associated hearing loss. Otolaryngcal Clin North Am. 2000;33:535-62.
16. Shin S, Guerra D, Rich M, Seung KJ, Mukherjee J, Joseph K, et al. Treatment of multidrug-resistant tuberculosis during pregnancy: a report of 7 cases. Clin Infect Dis. 2003;36:996-1003.
17. Swanson DS, Starke JR. Drug resistant tuberculosis in pediatrics. Pediatric Clinics of North America. 1995;42:553-81.
18. Takizawa T, Hashimoto K, Minami T, Yamashita S, Owen K. The comparative arthropathy of fluoroquinolones in dogs. Human and Experimental Toxicology. 1999;18:392-29.
19. Technical and Operational Guidelines for TB Control in India, 2016.
20. Valleho JG, Surke Jr. Tuberculosis and pregnancy. Clinic Chest Med. 1992;13:693-707.
21. World Health Organization. Treatment of TB Guidelines, 4th edition. WHO/HTM/TB/2009.420

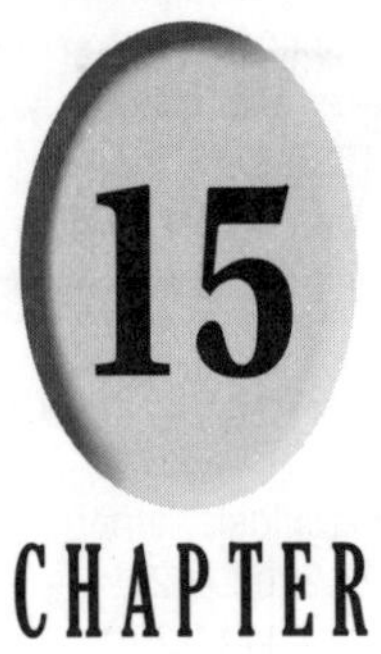

CHAPTER

Treatment of Multidrug Resistant Tuberculosis: Case-based Approach

CASE I

TS, a 18-year-old female diagnosed as pulmonary tuberculosis in 1995 and was prescribed rifampicin, isoniazid and ethambutol which she stopped herself after four months due to improvement. After five months of asymptomatic period, she again developed symptoms and prescribed rifampicin, isoniazid and ethambutol which she stopped after one month due to drug intolerance. Next time she received rifampicin, isoniazid, ethambutol and pyrazinamide in fix dose combination of controversial quality for next three months without any improvement. Thereafter treatment was changed to streptomycin, rifampicin, isoniazid, ethambutol and pyrazinamide for next two months, without any response. Then she received Category II treatment under RNTCP for nine months and still her sputum remained positive for AFB. In June 1997, she was hospitalized and her sputum was sent for culture and sensitivity for *Mycobacterium tuberculosis* and was treated with daily streptomycin, rifampicin, isoniazid, ethambutol and pyrazinamide in adequate doses under supervision. After four months of regular treatment her sputum remained positive for AFB. Her sputum culture and sensitivity report revealed resistance to rifampicin, isoniazid and streptomycin. Considering the past history of treatment, radiological, symptomatic deterioration and sensitivity report, she was diagnosed as MDR-TB. She was treated with injection kanamycin 0.75 g, PAS 10 g (in two divided doses), Ethionamide 500 mg and cycloserine 500 mg daily. 300 mg of isonizid was also given. Her sputum smear was examined every month for AFB. Kanamycin was stopped after 4 months when her sputum smear became negative for AFB. Rest of the treatment was continued for a period of 18 months. At the end of the treatment, sputum smear was negative for AFB and three cultures were negative for MTB. On subsequent follow-up for next five years, there was no relapse (Fig. 15.1).

CASE II

SS, a 15-year-old female, weighing 35 kg was diagnosed as a sputum positive new case of pulmonary tuberculosis in February 1998, with bad family history

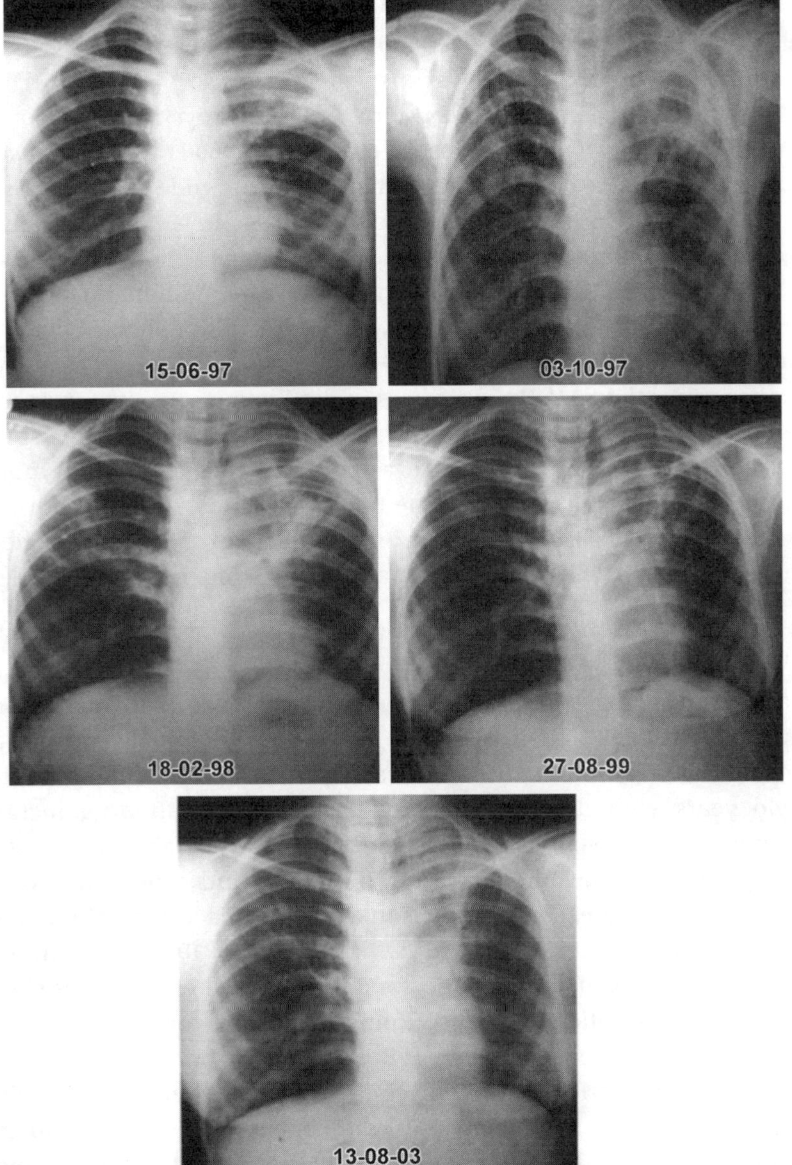

Fig. 15.1: Chest X-rays of case no I.

of her brother, who died of pulmonary tuberculosis after prolonged treatment for 4 years. She was prescribed 4 drug regimen comprising rifampicin, isoniazid, ethambutol and pyrazinamide in adequate doses, which she took regularly for 2 months, without any significant improvement clinically, radiologically as well as bacteriologically. Then she sought advice from other physician who added streptomycin and sparfloxacin to her previous regimen of 4 drugs. She took 6 drug regimens regularly for 6 months with negligible response clinically and radiologically. Subsequently she consulted us, when her sputum was positive for AFB and was also sent for culture and sensitivity for *Mycobacterium tuberculosis*. In light of her previous treatment experiences and outcomes, she was suspected as a case of primary MDR-TB. Pending sensitivity report, she was started on kanamycin 0.75 g, isoniazid 300 mg, PAS 8 g (in two divided doses), ethionamide 500 mg and cycloserine 500 mg daily in single dose. In September 1998 isoniazide 300 mg daily was also given. With the passage of time, she showed improvement clinically and radiologically, when her sputum became negative after 4 months. At the same time her sputum culture and sensitivity report from 4 different laboratories (sent at beginning of treatment) showed lots of discrepancies, with 2 of them labeling her as a case of MDR-TB while other labeling her as polydrug resistance other than MDR. Regardless of conflicting sensitivity reports we adhered to our regimen. Kanamycin was stopped after she became sputum negative, and rest of the treatment was continued for another 20 months. At the end of 2 years of treatment she was smear and culture negative with dramatic clearing of chest radiograph and weight gain of about 7 kg. She was followed for 5 years (till 2002), without any relapse (Fig. 15.2).

CASE III

MR, a 32-year-old male weighing 43 kg was diagnosed as a case of pulmonary tuberculosis in 1992 and was treated with 2 RHEZ/4 RHE and declared cured. He has relapsed in 1994 and was again treated by different doctors for two years with different inadequate regimens with drug including streptomycin, rifampicin, isoniazid, ethambutol and pyrazinamide without any response. He consulted another physician and took kanamycin (2 months), ethionamide, (2 months), isoniazid and thiacetazone for one year without any response. He came to us in September 1997 with complains of cough, fever, loss of appetite and weight. His serial chest X-rays showed progressive deterioration and his sputum was positive for AFB. Sputum was sent for culture and sensitivity for MTB. Pending the culture and sensitivity report, he was prescribed streptomycin, rifampicin, isoniazid, ethambutol and pyrazinamide in adequate doses with intensive health education. At the end of three months of regular treatment, he did not respond clinically and his sputum remained positive for AFB. Sputum culture (sent at the time of starting five drug) and sensitivity showed resistance to streptomycin, pyrazinamide, PAS and ethionamide with susceptibility to rifampicin, isoniazid, ethambutol, thiacetazone and cycloserine. However, in view of past history of ATT, his sensitivity report was ignored and was assumed as a case of MDR-TB and treatment was changed to injection kanamycin 0.75 g, PAS 10 g (in two divided doses), ethionamide 500 mg, pyrazinamide 1500 mg and ofloxacin 600 mg daily in December 1997, 300 mg of isonizid was also given. His sputum smear was examined for AFB every month. Patient developed

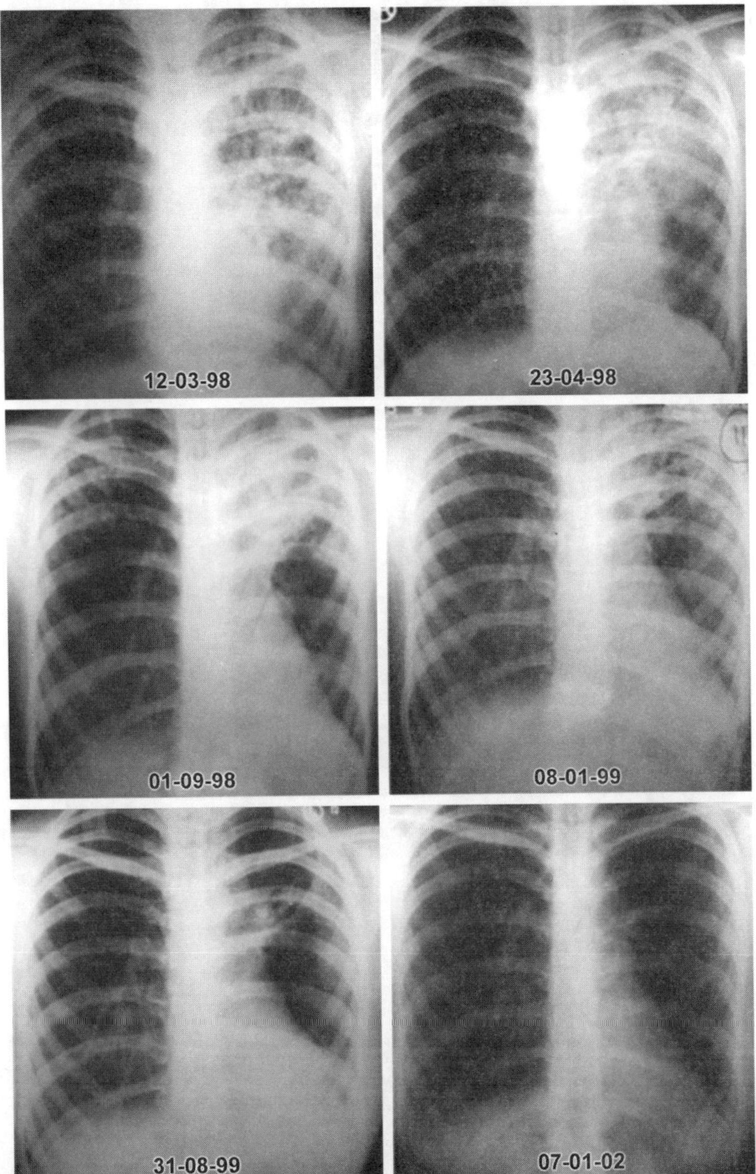

Fig. 15.2: Chest X-rays of case no II.

gastric intolerance in the beginning of treatment, however all the drugs were continued. Injection kanamycin was stopped after 6 months in June 1998 when his sputum became negative for AFB and rest of the drugs were continued for another 18 months. Patient responded clinically, radiologically and bacteriologically. Sputum smears for AFB and cultures were negative for MTB at the end of the treatment. Till now, after five years of regular follow up, he has not relapsed (Fig. 15.3).

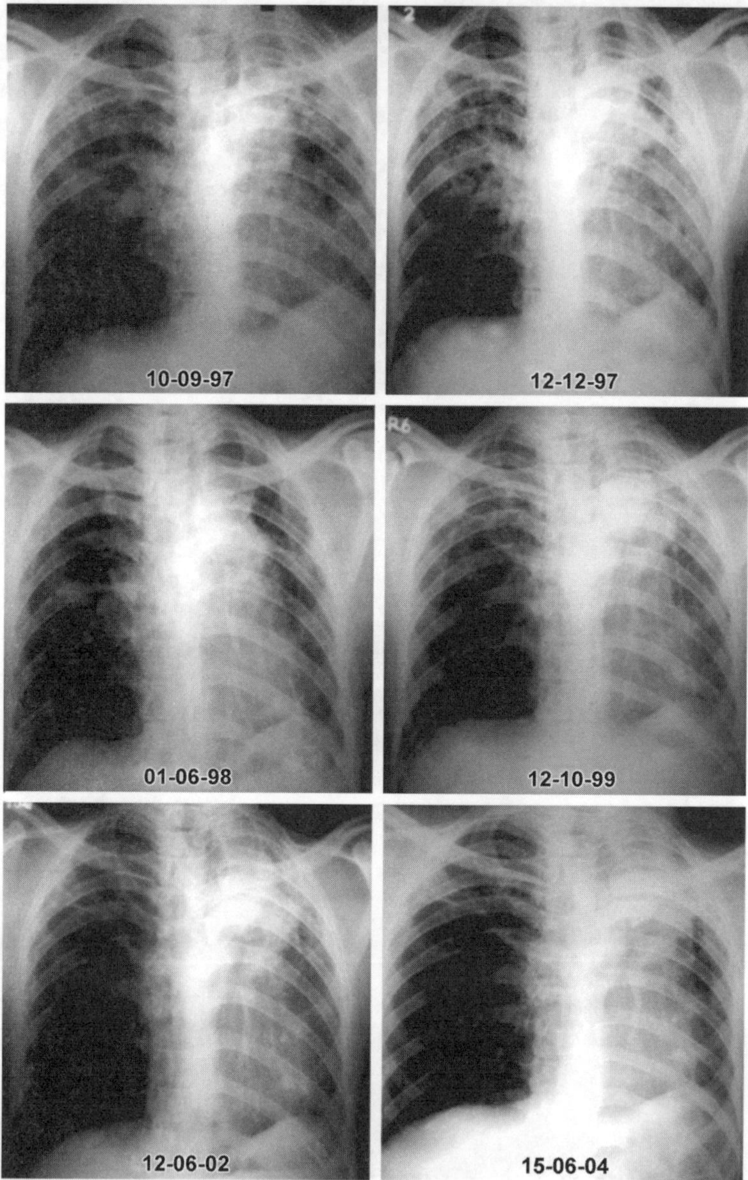

Fig. 15.3: Chest X-rays of case no III.

CASE IV

NK, a 27-year-male, weighing 40 kg presented with bilateral pulmonary tuberculosis with previous antitubercular treatment. Different doctors treated him for 4 years for pulmonary tuberculosis with different regimens in various combinations with drugs including streptomycin, isoniazid, rifampicin, ethambutol and pyrazinamide. His sputum was positive for AFB, which was sent for culture and sensitivity for *M. tuberculosis*. Pending culture report, treatment was started with five drug regimen of streptomycin 0.75 g, isoniazid 300 mg, rifampicin 450 mg, ethambutol 800 mg and pyrazinamide 1000 mg, daily in single dose, which he took regularly for 2 months without any clinical, radiological or bacteriological response. Sputum culture and sensitivity sent earlier, revealed drug resistance to streptomycin, isoniazid and rifampicin. On basis of this report, and previous history of treatment, he was kept on kanamycin 0.75 g, ethionamide 500 mg, ofloxacin 600 mg, ethambutol 800 mg and pyrazinamide 1000 mg daily in single dose. Isoniazid in single dose of 300 mg daily was also added. He responded clinically and bacteriologically, but his chest radiograph revealed no change on left side (which was destroyed), with some clearing of shadows in right lung. Sputum conversion occurred after 6 months of treatment, when kanamycin was stopped, and rest of drugs were continued for next 18 months. At the end of treatment, his sputum was negative for AFB and he has gained weight of 6 kg, but radiographical shadows persisted without much change, which in all likelihood will persist throughout his life and may be source of infection and hemoptysis in future (Fig. 15.4).

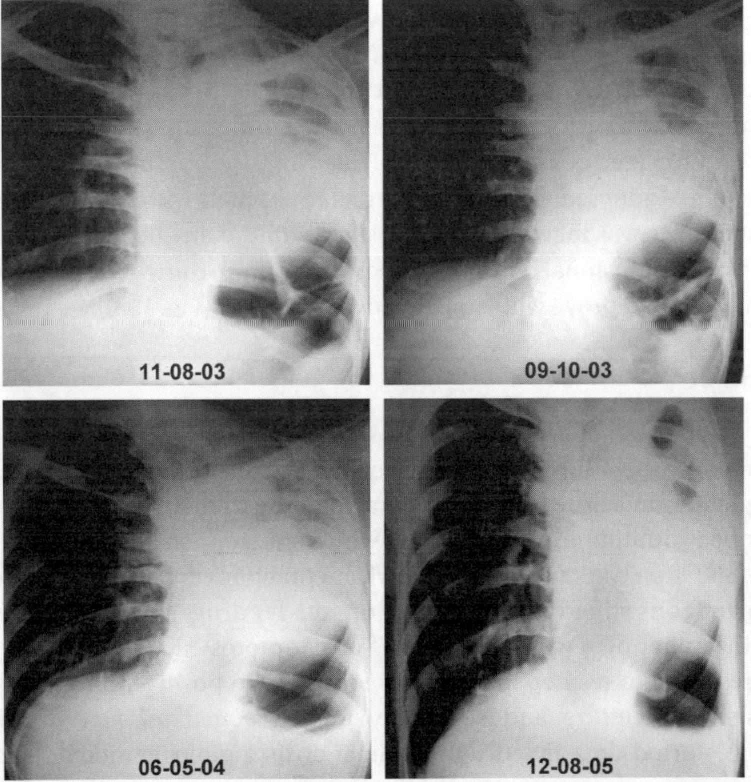

Fig. 15.4: Chest X-rays of case no IV.

CASE V

NR, a 35-year-male, weighing 40 kg, presented with bilateral pulmonary tuberculosis, with previous history of antitubercular treatment, from different doctors in various inadequate regimens, using streptomycin, isoniazid, rifampicin, ethambutol and pyrazinamide. At the time of presentation to us in January 2001, his sputum was positive for AFB, which was also sent for culture and sensitivity for *M. tuberculosis*. Pending sensitivity report, he was kept on regimen containing streptomycin 0.75 g, isoniazid 300 mg, rifampicin 450 mg, ethambutol 800 mg and pyrazinamide 1000 mg. Despite 4 months of regular treatment, there was no response on clinical, radiological and bacteriological parameters. Sputum culture and sensitivity sent at the beginning of treatment reported resistance to streptomycin, isoniazid, ethambutol and rifampicin. In light of this sensitivity report, previous inadequate treatment and lack of response to 4 months treatment of 5 drugs, he was diagnosed as a case of MDR TB, and kept on kanamycin 0.75 g, isoniazid 300 mg, PAS 8 g (in two divided doses), ethionamide 500 mg and cycloserine 500 mg daily in single dose. After one month of this therapy, he developed psychosis with suicidal tendency, which was managed by antipsychotic drugs, and cycloserine was replaced by ofloxacin 600 mg daily in single dose. His sputum became negative for AFB after 6 months of treatment, when kanamycin was stopped, and rest of drugs continued for next 18 months till April 2003, when he became smear and culture negative, and declared cured. While he was on this regimen, chest radiographic picture deteriorated, but sputum smear always remained negative. Considering this radiological deterioration as intercurrent pyogenic infection, we adhered to our antitubercular regimen with some appropriate antibiotics. He was followed up for 2 years, without any relapse, although he experienced occasional bouts of streaking of sputum during follow up period, which used to improve with conservative treatment (Fig. 15.5).

CASE VI

A 22-year-old female AV was diagnosed as a new case of sputum positive pulmonary tuberculosis in 2006. She was started on a regimen based on rifampicin, isoniazid, ethambutol, pyrazinamide from private practioner. She developed vomiting and gastritis after which she stopped her antituberculosis drugs. She then consulted multiple private practioners taking the prescribed treatment consisting of primary line of anti-TB drugs for 1–2 months then stopping at her own with partial relief of symptoms each time. In May 2008 she presented to us, her sputum was found to be positive for AFB, sputum was sent for culture and sensitivity for *Mycobacterial tuberculosis* and she was started on a five drug regimen consisting of rifampicin, isoniazid,

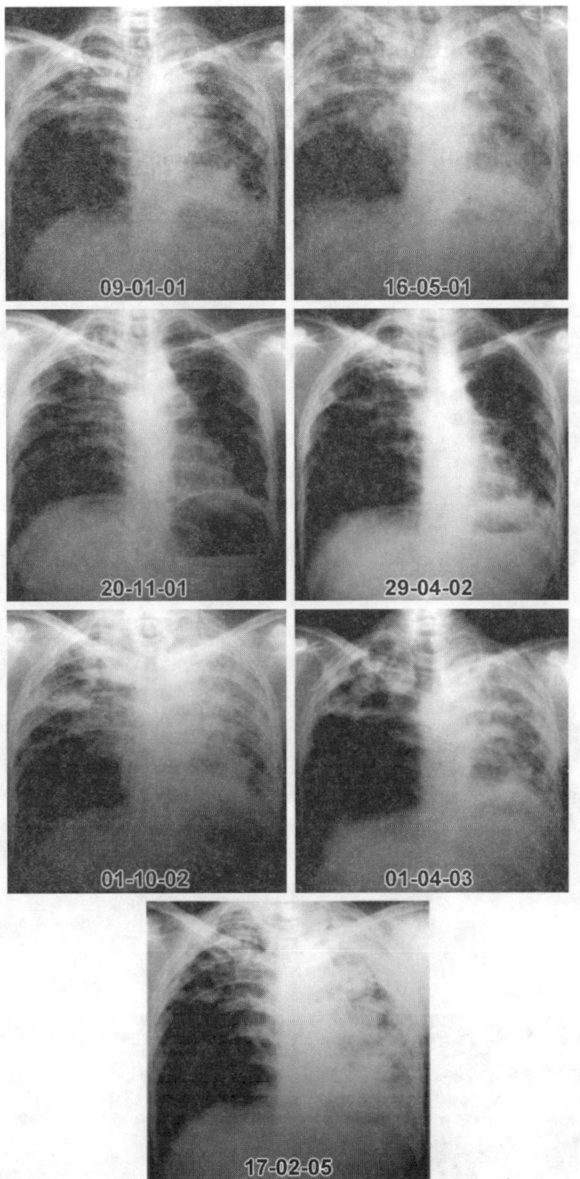

Fig. 15.5: Chest X-rays of case no V.

ethambutol, pyrazinamide and streptomycin. Her sputum culture sensitivity received in August 2008 showed growth of *Mycobacterium tuberculosis* which was resistant to rifampicin and isoniazid. She was started on regimen for MDR-TB consisting of injection kanamycin, pyrazinamide, ethambutol, ethionamide, cycloserine and ofloxacin. Her clinical condition improved, sputum for AFB and culture for *Mycobacterium* became negative 4th month onwards. Kanamycin and pyrazinamide were stopped after 6 months. Rest of the treatment was continued for 18 months. Patient responded clinically, radiologically and bacteriologically. Sputum and culture were negative for *Mycobacterium tuberculosis* at the end of treatment in 2010. On subsequent follow up for two years she was asymptomatic (Fig. 15.6).

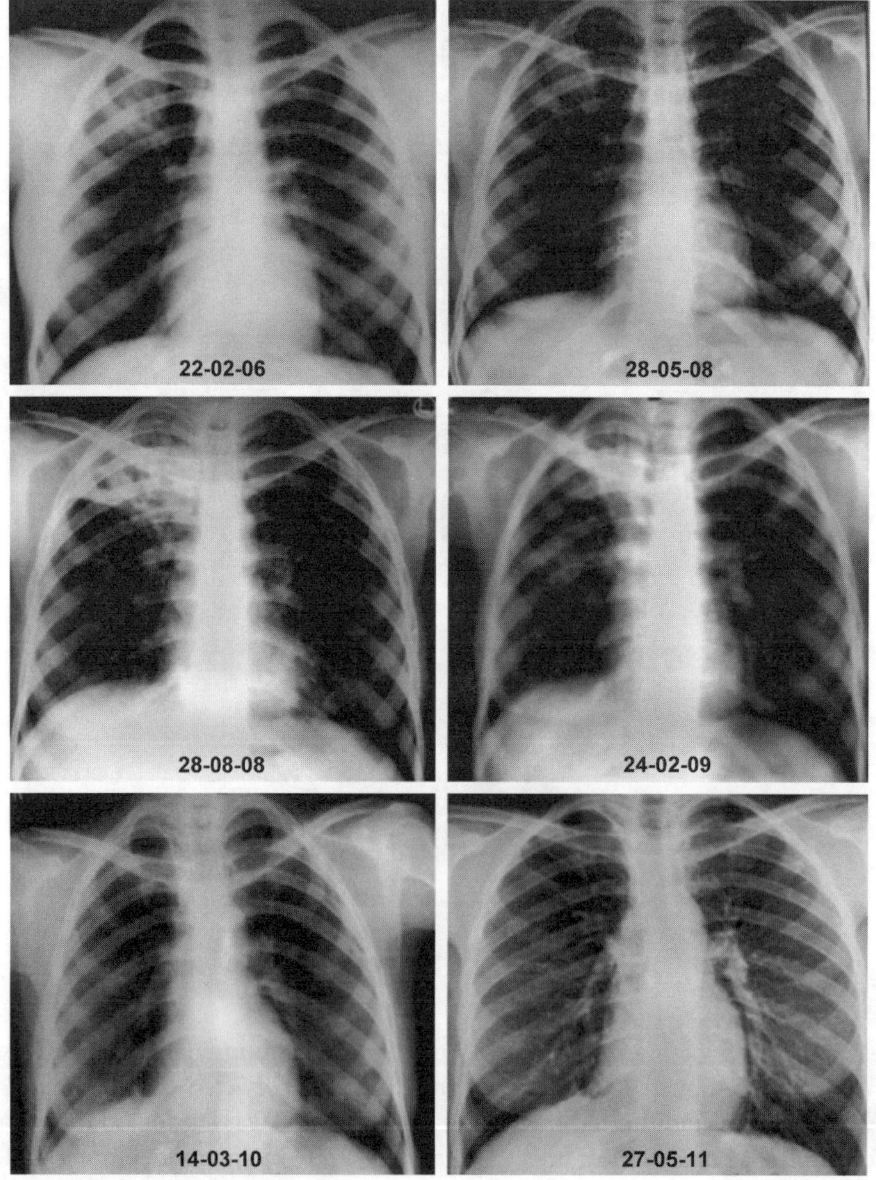

Fig. 15.6: Chest X-rays of case no VI.

CASE VII

A 21-year-old male presented with chief complains of fever since 1 month, loss of weight and loss of appetite. Patient was started on a regimen based on rifampicin, isoniazid, pyrazinamide and ethambutol by private practitioner which he took for 7 months but patient continued to have fever and there was no resolution of chest infiltrates. Patient was referred to our center in November 2014. Gene Xpert in December 2014 detected rifampicin resistance. His culture sensitivity showed resistance to isoniazid, rifampicin, pyrazinamide, ethambutol, streptomycin, ciprofloxacin and was susceptible to kanamycin, levofloxacin, amikacin, capreomycin. Patient was put on a regimen for MDR-TB in December 2014 consisting of kanamycin, ethionamide, cycloserine, levofloxacin, pyrazinamide and ethambutol. Kanamycin was stopped at 9 months when sputum smear and culture for MTB became negative. Rest of the drugs including pyrazinamide were continued for 20 months. It is worth to note that pyrazinamide were given throughout the treatment. Patient sputum smear and culture remained negative for *Mycobacterium tuberculosis*. There was significant improvement clinically and radiologically. Patient remained asymptomatic after 6 months of follow up after stopping the treatment.

CASE VIII

A 17-year-old female presented with chief complains of fever since 1 month, loss of weight and loss of appetite. Her sputum smear for AFB was positive and was given a regimen containing rifampicin, isoniazid, pyrazinamide and ethambutol by private practitioner which she took for 12 months but patient continued to have fever and there was no resolution of chest infiltrates. Patient was referred to our center in December 2015. Her sputum smear was positive for AFB in December inspite of 12 months of antitubercular treatment. Patient was started on a five drug regimen containing rifampicin, isoniazid, pyrazinamide, ethambutol and streptomycin pending culture and drug susceptibility (DST) report. Gene Xpert detected rifampicin resistance in December 2015. Her culture and susceptibility report showed resistance to isoniazid, kanamycin, ofloxacin and was susceptible to moxifloxacin, capreomycin. Though the DST showed XDR-TB but the patient has never received kanamycin and ofloxacin so patient was put on a regimen for MDR-TB in February 2016 containing kanamycin, ethionamide, cycloserine, ethambutol, pyrazinamide and moxifloxacin. Kanamycin was stopped at 9 months when sputum smear and culture for MTB became negative.

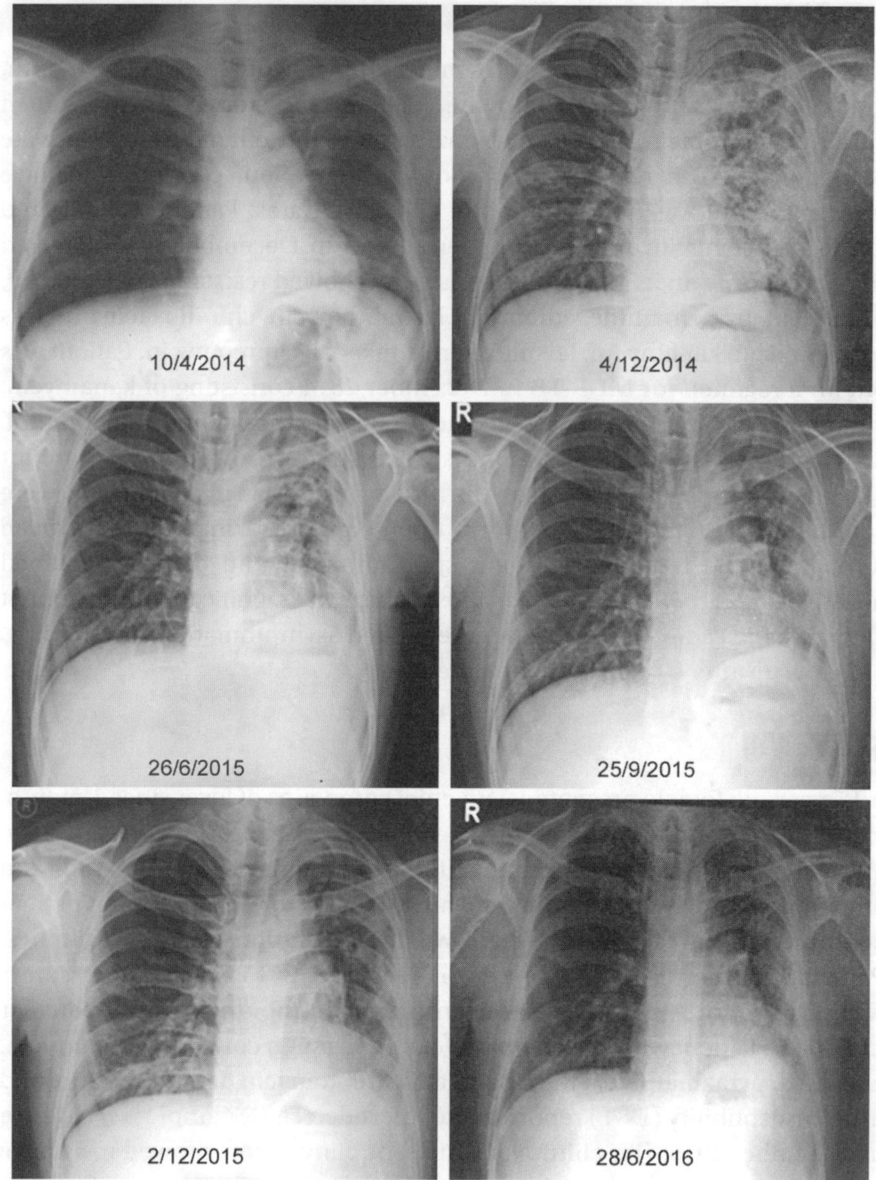

Fig. 15.7: Chest X-rays of case no VII.

Rest of the drugs were continued. It is worth to note that pyrazinamide was given throughout the treatment. Patient sputum smear and culture became negative for mycobacterium tuberculosis. There was significant improvement clinically and radiologically. Patient is still on treatment.

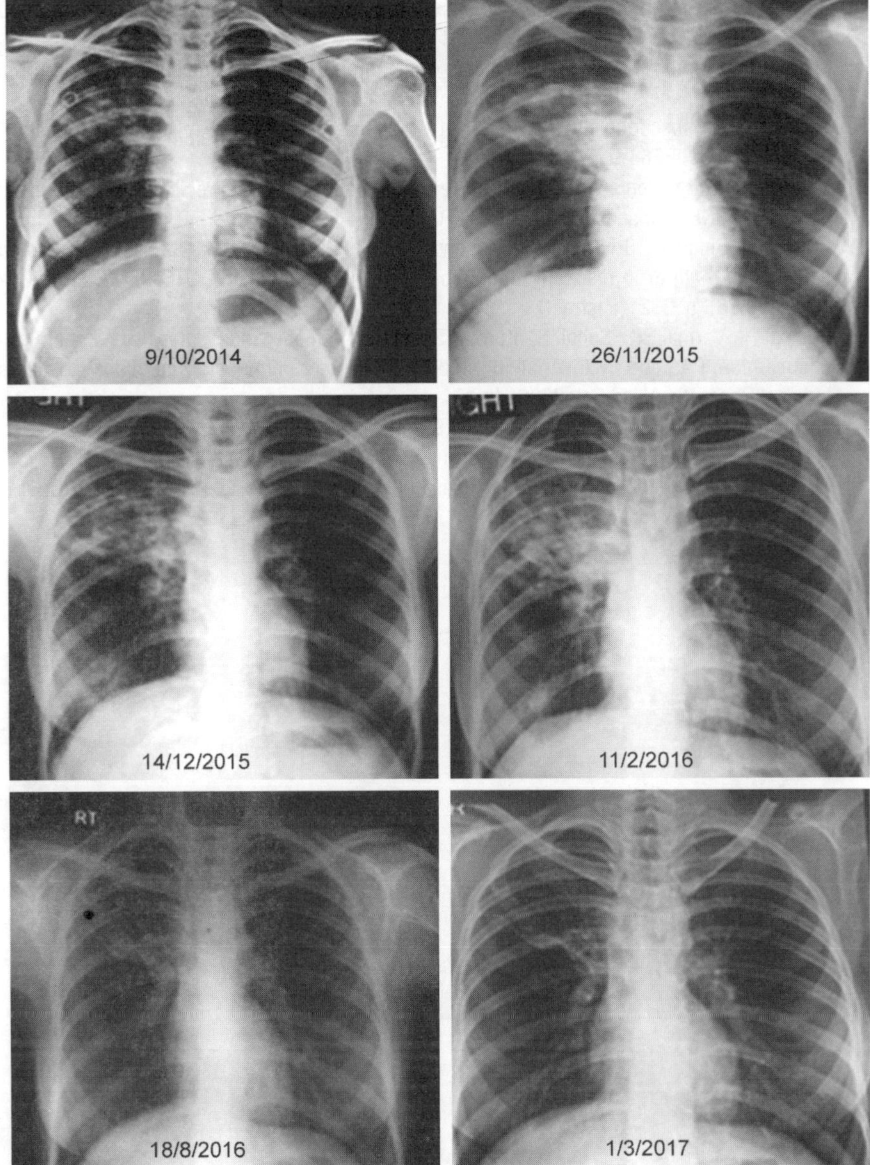

Fig. 15.8: Chest X-rays of case no VIII.

FURTHER READINGS

1. Caminero JA. Management of multidrug-resistant tuberculosis and patients in retreatment. Eur Respir J. 2005; 25: 928-36.
2. Companion Handbook to the WHO guidelines for the programmatic management of drug resistant tuberculosis. WHO/HTM/TB/2014.11

3. Guidelines for programmatic management of drug resistant tuberculosis. WHO, 2011. WHO/HTM/TB/2011.6
4. International Union Against Tuberculosis and Lung Diseases. Guidelines for Clinical and Operational Management of Drug-Resistant Tuberculosis. IUTLD, Paris; 2013.
5. Kim SJ. Drug susceptibility testing in tuberculosis: methods and reliability of results. E Respir J. 2005;25:564-9.
6. Management of patients with multidrug resistant/extensively drug-resistant tuberculosis in Europe: a TBNET consensus statement. ERJ. 2014; 44:23-63.
7. Prasad R, Singh A, Srivastava R, Kushwaha RAS, Garg R, Verma SK, et al. Treatment outcome of multi drug resistant tuberculosis patients in modified DOTS PLUS. ERJ 2012; 40, (suppl56): p. 3321(abstract)
8. Prasad R, Verma SK, Sahai S, Kumar S, Jain A. Efficacy and safety of Kanamycin, Ethionamide, PAS and cycloserine in multi drug resistant pulmonary tuberculosis patients. Indian J Chest Dis Allied Sci. 2006; 48:181-4.
9. Technical and Operational Guidelines for TB Control in India, 2016.
10. Treatment of Tuberculosis: Guidelines, 4th edition. WHO\HTM\TB\2009.420.
11. WHO treatment guidelines for Drug-Resistent Tuberculosis – 2016 Update. WHO/HTM/TB/2016.04.

CHAPTER 16 Shorter Regimen to Treat Multidrug Resistant Tuberculosis and Rifampicin Resistant TB

Multidrug resistant tuberculosis (MDR-TB), defined as disease due to *Mycobacterium tuberculosis* that is resistant to at least both rifampicin and isoniazid with or without other anti-tuberculosis (TB) drugs or rifampicin resistant TB (RR-TB) defined as resistance to rifampicin detected using genotypic or phenotypic methods with or without resistance to other anti-TB drugs is emerging as major problem due to poor management of drug sensitive as well as drug resistance TB. MDR-TB is treatable but is very expensive, requires long duration of treatment (usually 2 years) and contains potentially toxic drugs. The Global Tuberculosis Report 2016 estimated that of 3.9% newly diagnosed and 21% of previously treated tuberculosis cases had MDR-TB. It has been estimated that 580,000 cases of TB resistant to at least rifampicin (RR-TB) globally in 2015 of whom 480,000 were having resistant to both rifampicin and isoniazid (MDR-TB) and 250,000 death occurred due to MDR-TB/RR-TB in 2015 globally. Out of estimated 580,000 MDR-TB/RR-TB cases, only 132120 (23%) were detected and even fewer 124990 (20%) started treatment and only 52% of them were treated successfully. In India, estimates showed that the prevalence of MDR-TB among new and previously treated patients was 2.5% and 16% respectively. It is estimated that 130,000 cases of MDR-TB/RR-TB emerged in India of which 79,000 were among notified cases of TB in 2015. Out of 79000 MDR–TB cases, only 28,876 were diagnosed, 26,988 were started on treatment and treatment success rate was only 46%. The reasons for poor result are probably due to lengthy, expensive and toxic regimens leading to poor compliance.

WHO update 2016 for drug resistant TB has introduced a shorter regimen treatment for MDR-TB/RR-TB which aims to reduce cost, improve compliance and cure rate. In patients with rifampicin-resistant TB (RR-TB) or multidrug-resistant TB who has not been previously treated with second-line drugs and in whom resistance to flouroquinolones and second-line injectable agents has been excluded or is considered highly unlikely, a shorter MDR-TB regimen of 9–12 months may be used instead of a conventional regimen of usually two years duration. Shorter MDR regimen consists of intensive phase of 4

TABLE 16.1: Drugs and doses used in shorter MDR-TB regimen.

Product	Weight group		
	<33 kg	33–50 kg	>50 kg
Moxifloxacin	400 mg	600 mg	800 mg
Clofazimine	50 mg	100 mg	100 mg
Ethambutol	800 mg	800 mg	1,200 mg
Pyrazinamide	1,000 mg	1,500 mg	2,000 mg
Isoniazid	300 mg	400 mg	600 mg
Prothionamide	250 mg	500 mg	750 mg
Kanamycin	15 mg per kilogram body weight (maximum 1 g)		

months (extended to 6 months in case of lack of sputum smear conversion) containing gatifloxacin or moxifloxacin, kanamycin, prothionamide, clofazimine, high-dose isoniazid, pyrazinamide, and ethambutol followed by a continuation phase of 5 months containing gatifloxacin or moxifloxacin, clofazimine, ethambutol, and pyrazinamide. Doses of each drug in shorter MDR-TB regimen are given in Table 16.1.

It can be given to children, adults and people living with HIV who meet above specified criteria but should not be used in extrapulmonary TB and in pregnant females. This recommendation is based on meta-analysis of results of initial programmatic studies conducted by the Union, Damien Foundation, Medicines Sans Frontiers (MSF) and the Antwerp Institute of Tropical Medicine in Belgium, involving 1205 patients with the uncomplicated MDR-TB. Data of 515 patients under the Damien Foundation pilot programmer, using a 9 month treatment regimen in Bangladesh, showed cure rate of 82.1% and overall success rate of 84.5%. Whether the shorter MDR-TB regimen will work in all settings and especially outside trial conditions is to be seen. However, the fundamentals of the shorter regimen are practically the same as conventional 24 months treatment. Shorter regimen is using the same number of drugs including flourquinolones, a second-line injectable and two other drugs. The only difference is that fluoroquinolone used is gatifloxacin/moxifloxacin instead of levofloxacin and replacement of cycloserine with clofazimine. This study was followed by the Union coordinated first multi-country MDR-TB patient cohort study of 1,000 patients in 9 countries of West Africa (Benin, Burkina-Faso, Burundi, Cameroon, Côte d'Ivoire, Central African Republic, Niger, Democratic Republic of Congo and Rwanda), treated with a modified Bangladesh regimen. Interim analysis of 408 patients has reported 82.1% treatment success rate, demonstrating that the 9 month regimen can be successful in other environments than Bangladesh, and also in settings with high HIV prevalence. They showed shorter MDR-TB treatment regimens given in patents who met specific inclusion criteria had a statistically-significant higher likelihood of treatment success than those who received longer conventional regimens (89.9% vs. 78.3%). It will improve adherence, drug safety and tolerability. It will also reduce the cost to approximately half of the conventional MDR-TB Regimen. Shorter MDR-TB regimen will be the useful tool in the fight against MDR/XDR-TB if properly utilized.

Question arises in mind whether, programmatic management of MDR-TB with a shorter regimen will lead to XDR-TB. Currently, there is no evidence for this as shorter regimen has produced excellent results under the operational research conditions in some settings. Shorter MDR-TB regimen will allow for more patients to be treated, more chance of completing treatment and ultimately will reduce the number of MDR and XDR-TB patients over the time. Currently, the strongest risk for unfavorable outcome with shorter regimen is high level fluoroquinolone resistance especially when associated with initial pyrazinamide resistance. If resistance is present for one or more drugs in the shorter regimen then possibly, these could be replaced with linezolid, delamanid or bedaquiline and still maintain shorter treatment duration. However, there is no sufficient evidence to recommend this. Resistance to pyrazinamide even if evident by reliable drug susceptibility testing (DST) is not an absolute contraindication for the shorter regimen; unless there are indications that one or other drugs in the regimen are also resistant. It is not recommended to base treatment decision as DST for ethambutol owing to unreliable DST results and there is no reliable DST available for clofazimine or prothionamide at present. Currently, Union-sponsored and USAID supported STREAM stage1 study (multi-center international randomized controlled trial) which was started in July 2012 to evaluate shortened regimens for patients with MDR-TB is underway and results are expected in 1st quarter of 2018. STREAM has recently expanded (stage 2) to test two additional shorter treatment regimens using bedaquiline. This expanded arm will evaluate a 9 month all-oral regimen without injections and an even shorter simplified 6-month regimen. It will finish enrollment of patients in 2018 and initial results are expected by 2020. New hope on the new, shorter and successful treatment for MDR-TB is now with us especially in high burden countries including India.

FURTHER READINGS

1. Ahuja SD, Ashkin D, Avendano M, Banerjee R, Bauer M, Bayona JN, et al. Multidrug resistant pulmonary tuberculosis treatment regimens and patient outcomes: an individual patient data meta-analysis of 9,153 patients. PLoS Med. 2012;9:e1001300.
2. Aung KJ,Van Deun A,Declercq E et al. Successful '9-month Bangaldesh regimen'for multidrug resistant tuberculosis among over 500 consecutive patients.Int J Tubec Lung Dis. 2014;18:1180-87.

3. Companion Handbook to the WHO guidelines for the programmatic management of drug resistant tuberculosis. WHO/HTM/TB/2014.11
4. Kuaban C, Noeske J, Rieder HL, Aït-Khaled N, Abena Foe JL, Trébucq A. High effectiveness of a 12-month regimen for MDR-TB patients in Cameroon. Int J Tuberc Lung Dis Off J Int Union Tuberc Lung Dis. 2015 ;19:517-24.
5. Nunn AJ, Rusen ID, Van Deun A, et al. Evaluation of a standardized treatment regimen of anti-tuberculosis drugs for patients with multi-drug-resistant tuberculosis (STREAM): study protocol for a randomized controlled trial. Trials. 2014;15:353.
6. Piubello A, Harouna SH, Souleymane MB, Boukary I, Morou S, Daouda M, et al. High cure rate with standardised short-course multidrug-resistant tuberculosis treatment in Niger: no relapses. Int J Tuberc Lung Dis. 2014 ;18:1188-94.
7. Prasad R, Gupta N, Singh M. Multidrug resistant tuberculosis: trends and control. Indian J Chest Dis Allied Sci. 2014; 56: 237-46.
8. Prasad R, Gupta N. MDR & XDR tuberculosis. In: Multidrug resistant Tuberculosis: Diagnosis and Treatment, 1st edition. New Delhi: Jaypee Brothers Medical Publisher (P) Ltd. 2015: pp. 92-111.
9. Prasad R, Srivastava DK. Multidrug and Extensively drug resistant TB (M/XDR TB) management: Current issues. Clinical Epidemiology and Global Health. 2013;1:124-8.
10. Prasad R. Multidrug and extensively drug-resistant tuberculosis management: evidences and controversies. Lung India. 2012;29:154-9.
11. Trébucq A, Schwoebel V, Kuaban C, et al. Expanding shortened MDR-TB treatment: the West African experience. Int J Tuberc Lung Dis. 2014;18(Suppl):S15.
12. Van Deun A, Maug AKJ, Salim MAH, Das PK, Sarker MR, Daru P, et al. Short, highly effective, and inexpensive standardized treatment of multidrug-resistant tuberculosis. Am J Respir Crit Care Med. 2010;182:684-9.
13. WHO treatment guidelines for drug-resistant tuberculosis 2016 update. WHO/HTM/TB/2016.04.
14. World Health Organization. Global Tuberculosis Report. 2016.WHO/HTM/2016.13.Geneva World Health Organization; 2016.

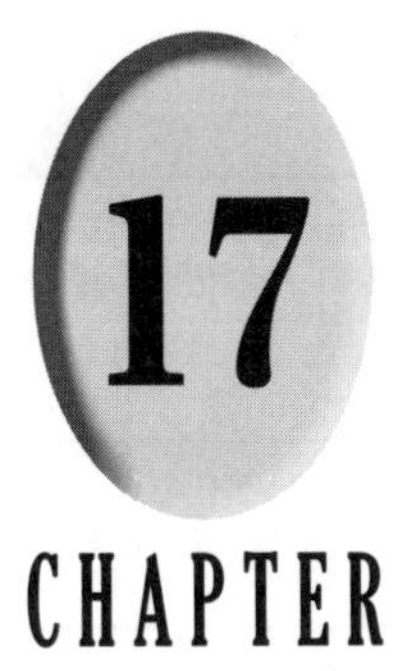

CHAPTER

Monitoring of Treatment and Adverse Drug Reactions in Drug Resistant Tuberculosis

The initial evaluation serves to establish a baseline and may identify patients who are at increased risk for adverse effects or poor outcomes. The monitoring of treatment and the management of adverse effects may have to be more intensive in patients with pre-existing conditions or conditions identified at the initial evaluation (diabetes mellitus, renal insufficiency, acute or chronic liver disease, thyroid disease, mental illness, drug or alcohol dependence, HIV infection, pregnancy, lactation and others). This review aims to addresses the monitoring requirements for the treatment of drug resistant tuberculosis (DR-TB), adverse effects associated with different second-line drugs, strategies for the early detection and treatment of adverse effects and also adverse effects in human immunodeficiency virus (HIV) coinfected patients with DR-TB.

PRETREATMENT SCREENING AND EVALUATION

The required initial pretreatment clinical investigation includes a thorough medical history and physical examination. The recommended initial evaluation and monitoring during treatment of DR-TB are shown in Table 17.1.

TABLE 17.1: Pretreatment evaluation and monitoring during DR-TB treatment.

Monitoring evaluation	Recommended frequency
Evaluation by clinician	At baseline, and at least monthly until conversion, then every 2–3 months
Sputum smears and cultures	For follow-up examination four sputum specimens will be collected and examined by smear and culture at least 30 days apart from the 3rd to 7th month of treatment (i.e. at the end of the months 3, 4, 5, 6 and 7) and at 3-monthly intervals from the 9th month onwards till the completion of treatment (i.e. at the end of the months 9, 12, 15, 18, 21 and 24)
Weight	At baseline and then monthly

Contd...

Contd...

Monitoring evaluation	Recommended frequency
Drug susceptibility	At baseline to confirm MDR-TB. For patients who remain culture-positive, it is not necessary to repeat DST within less than 3 months of treatment
Chest radiograph	At baseline, and then every 6 months
Serum creatinine	At baseline, then monthly if possible while receiving an injectable drug. Every 1–3 weeks in HIV-infected patients, diabetes and other high-risk patients
Serum potassium	Monthly while receiving an injectable agent. Every 1–3 weeks in HIV-infected patients, diabetics and other high-risk patients
Serum magnesium and calcium	Check magnesium and calcium blood levels whenever hypokalaemia is diagnosed. At baseline and then monthly if on bedaquiline or delamanid. Repeat if any electrocardiogram (ECG) abnormalities develop (prolonged QT interval)
Thyroid-stimulating hormone (TSH)	Every 6 months if receiving ethionamide/prothionamide and/or PAS; and monitor monthly for signs/symptoms of hypothyroidism. TSH is sufficient for screening for hypothyroidism; it is not necessary to measure hormone thyroid levels
Liver serum enzymes	Periodic monitoring (every 1–3 months) in patients receiving pyrazinamide for extended periods or for patients at risk for or with symptoms of hepatitis. For HIV-infected patients, do monthly monitoring For patients on bedaquiline, monitor monthly. For patients with viral hepatitis, monitor every one to two weeks for the first month and then every one to four weeks
HIV screening	At baseline, and repeat if clinically indicated
Pregnancy tests	At baseline for women of childbearing age, and repeat if indicated
Hemoglobin and white blood count	If on linezolid, monitor weekly at first, then monthly or as needed based on symptoms; there is little clinical experience with prolonged use. For HIV-positive patients on an ART regime that includes AZT, monitor monthly initially and then as needed, based on symptoms
Lipase	Indicated for work up of abdominal pain to rule out pancreatitis in patients on linezolid, stavudine, didanosine and zalcitabine
Lactic acidosis	Indicated for work up of lactic acidosis in patients on linezolid or antiretroviral treatment
Serum glucose	If receiving gatifloxacin, monitor glucose frequently (weekly) and educate patient on signs and symptoms of hypoglycemia and hyperglycemia
Audiometry	Baseline audiogram and then monthly while on an injectable agent. Ask patients about changes in hearing at every clinic visit and evaluate their ability to participate in normal conversation

Contd...

Contd...

Monitoring evaluation	Recommended frequency
Vision tests	For patients on long-term ethambutol or linezolid perform at least a visual acuity test with Snellen charts and colour vision test at baseline (as a small percentage of the population has colour blindness). Repeat the test for any suspicion of change in acuity or colour vision
Educational, psychological and social consultation	At baseline by personnel trained in health education, psychological and social issues relevant to TB management; during treatment and repeat as indicated. Refer to social worker, psychologist or psychiatrist when indicated
Electrocardiography (ECG)	An ECG should be obtained before initiation of treatment with bedaquiline or delamanid, and at least 2, 4, 8, 12, and 24 weeks after starting treatment. Monitoring ECGs should be done monthly if taking other QT prolonging drugs (i.e moxifloxacin, clofazimine)

MONITORING PROGRESS OF TREATMENT

Clinically, the most important way to monitor response to treatment is through regular history taking and physical examination. The classic symptoms of TB like cough, sputum production, fever and weight loss generally improve within the first few months of treatment and should be monitored frequently by health-care providers. Patients should be monitored closely for signs of treatment failure. The recurrence of TB symptoms after sputum conversion, for example, may be the first sign of treatment failure. For children, height and weight should be measured regularly to ensure that they are growing normally. A normal growth rate should resume after a few months of successful treatment. Objective laboratory evidence of improvement often lags behind clinical improvement. The chest radiograph may be unchanged or show only slight improvement, especially in retreatment patients with chronic pulmonary lesions. Chest radiographs should be taken at least every six months, when a surgical intervention is being considered, or whenever the patient's clinical situation has worsened. The most important objective evidence of improvement is conversion of the sputum smear and culture to negative. While sputum smear is still useful clinically because of its much shorter turnaround time. Sputum culture is much more sensitive and is necessary to monitor the progress of treatment. Sputum examinations are also dependent on the quality of the sputum produced, so care should be taken to obtain adequate specimens. Persistently positive sputum and cultures for *Mycobacterium tuberculosis* bacilli should be assessed for nontuberculous mycobacteria (NTM), as overgrowth with NTM in lung damage secondary to TB is not uncommon. In such cases, although DR-TB may be adequately treated, treatment may need to be directed towards the NTM as well sputum conversion is slower in DR-TB than in drug-susceptible TB. Paucibacillary culture results should not be automatically regarded as negative when treating DR-TB. Acquired drug resistance and treatment failure often begin with the growth of one or two colonies on a sputum culture. Culture conversion should not be considered to be equivalent to cure. A certain proportion of patients may initially convert and later revert to positive sputum culture. Sputum smears and cultures should be monitored closely throughout treatment. These guidelines recommend that the tests should be performed monthly before smear and culture conversion, with conversion defined as two consecutive negative smears and cultures taken 30 days apart. After conversion, the minimum period recommended for bacteriological monitoring is monthly for smears and quarterly for cultures. Programs with adequate culture capacity may choose to do cultures more frequently, every 1–2 months, after conversion. Specimens for monitoring do not need to be examined in duplicate, but doing so can increase the sensitivity of the monitoring. For patients who remain smear- and culture-positive during treatment or who are suspects for treatment failure, drug susceptibility testing (DST) can be repeated. It is usually not necessary to repeat DST within less than three months of completion of treatment.

MONITORING FOR ADVERSE EFFECTS DURING TREATMENT

Close monitoring of patients is necessary to ensure that the adverse effects of second-line drugs are recognized quickly by health-care worker. The ability to monitor patients for adverse effects daily is one of the major advantages of directly observed therapy (DOT) over self-administration of DR-TB treatment. The majority of adverse effects are easy to recognize. Commonly, patients will volunteer that they are experiencing adverse effects. However, it is important to have a systematic method of patient interviewing since some patients may not reveal even severe adverse effects. Other patients may be distracted by one adverse effect and forget to tell the health-care provider about others. Laboratory screening is invaluable for detecting certain adverse effects that are more occult .The recommendations based on the experience of several PMDT projects for the minimal frequency of essential laboratory screening is given in Table 17.1. More frequent screening may be advisable, particularly for high-risk patients. Nephrotoxicity is a known complication of the injectable drugs, both of aminoglycosides and of capreomycin. This adverse effect is occult in onset and can be fatal. The optimal timing for checking serum creatinine is unknown, but most current treatment programs for DR-TB check serum creatinine at least monthly. In addition, patients with a history of renal disease (including comorbidities such as HIV and diabetes), advanced age or any renal symptoms should be monitored more closely, particularly at the start of treatment. An estimate of the glomerular filtration rate may help to further stratify the risk of nephrotoxicity in these patients. Electrolyte imbalance is a known complication of the antituberculosis injectable drugs, most frequently with capreomycin. It is generally a late effect occurring after months of treatment, and is reversible once the injectable drug is suspended. Since electrolyte imbalance is often occult in the early stages and can be easily managed with electrolyte replacement, serum potassium should be checked at least monthly in high-risk patients, and in all those taking capreomycin. Hypothyroidism is a late effect provoked by PAS and ethionamide. It is suspected by clinical assessment and confirmed by testing the serum level of thyroid-stimulating hormone (TSH). The use of these agents together can produce hypothyroidism in up to 10% of patients. Since the symptoms can be subtle, it is recommended that patients are screened for hypothyroidism with a serum TSH at 6–9 months, and then tested again every 6 months or sooner if symptoms arise. The dosing of thyroid replacement therapy should be guided using serum levels of TSH. Goiters can develop due to the toxic effects of PAS, ethionamide or prothionamide.

MANAGEMENT OF ADVERSE EFFECTS

Second-line drugs have many more adverse effects than the first-line antituberculosis drugs. Proper management of adverse effects begins with patient education. Before starting treatment, the patient should be instructed in detail about the potential adverse effects that could be produced by the prescribed drug regimen. Prompt evaluation, diagnosis and treatment of adverse effects are extremely important, even if the adverse effect is not particularly dangerous. Patients may have significant fear and anxiety about an adverse effect if they do not understand why it is happening. These emotions in turn may augment the severity of the adverse effect, as in the case of nausea and vomiting. If the adverse effect is mild and not dangerous, continuing the treatment regimen, with the help of ancillary drugs if needed, is often the best option. In patients with highly resistant TB, a satisfactory replacement drug may not be available, so that suspending a drug will make the treatment regimen less potent. Some adverse effects may disappear or diminish with time, and patients may be able to continue receiving the drug if sufficiently motivated. The adverse effects of a number of second-line drugs are highly dose dependent. Reducing the dosage of the offending drug is another method of managing adverse effects, but only in cases where the reduced dose is still expected to produce adequate serum levels and not compromise the regimen. With cycloserine and ethionamide, for example, a patient may be completely intolerant at one dose and completely tolerant at a slightly lower dose. Unfortunately, given the narrow therapeutic margins of these drugs, lowering the dose may also affect efficacy, so every effort should be made to maintain an adequate dose of the drug according to body weight.

Pyridoxine (vitamin B_6) should be given to all patients receiving cycloserine or terizidone to help prevent neurological adverse effects. The recommended dose is 50 mg for every 250 mg of cycloserine (or terizidone) prescribed. Psychosocial support is an important component of the management of adverse effects. The common adverse effects, the likely responsible antituberculosis agents and the suggested management strategies are given in Table 17.2.

TABLE 17.2: Common adverse effects, suspected agent(s) and management strategies of antituberculous drugs used in drug resistant TB.

Adverse effect	Suspected agent	Suggested management strategies
Seizures	**CS** H Fq	• Suspend suspected agent pending resolution of seizures • Initiate anticonvulsant therapy (e.g. phenytoin, valproic acid) • Increase pyridoxine to maximum daily dose (200 mg per day) • Restart suspected agent or reinitiate suspected agent at lower dose, if essential to the regimen • Discontinue suspected agent if this can be done without compromising regimen • Anticonvulsant is generally continued until MDR-TB treatment is completed or suspected agent discontinued • History of previous seizure disorder is not a contraindication to the use of agents listed here if a patient's seizures are well controlled and/or the patient is receiving anticonvulsant • Patients with history of previous seizures may be at increased risk for development of seizures during MDR-TB treatment
Peripheral neuropathy	**CS** **Lzd** **H** S Km Am Cm Eto/Pto Fq	• Increase pyridoxine to maximum daily dose (200 mg per day) • Change injectable to capreomycin if patient has documented susceptibility to capreomycin • Initiate therapy with tricyclic antidepressants such as amitriptyline. Non-steroidal anti-inflammatory drugs or acetaminophen may help alleviate symptoms • Lower dose of suspected agent, if this can be done without compromising regimen • Discontinue suspected agent if this can be done without compromising regimen • Patients with comorbid disease, e.g. diabetes, HIV, alcohol neuropathy (dependence) may be more likely to develop peripheral neuropathy, but these conditions are not contraindications to the use of the agents • Neuropathy may be irreversible; however, some patients may experience improvement when offending agents are suspended
Hearing loss	**S** **Km** **Am** **Cm** Clr	• Document hearing loss and compare with baseline audiometry if available • Change parenteral treatment to capreomycin if patient has documented susceptibility to capreomycin

(Contd.)

(Contd.)

Adverse effect	Suspected agent	Suggested management strategies
		• Decrease frequency and/or lower dose of suspected agent if this can be done without compromising the regimen (consider administration three times per week) • Discontinue suspected agent if this can be done without compromising the regimen • Patients with previous exposure to aminoglycosides may have baseline hearing loss. In such patients, audiometry may be helpful at the start of MDR-TB treatment • Hearing loss is generally not reversible • The risk of further hearing loss must be weighed against the risks of stopping the injectable in the treatment regimen • While the benefit of hearing aids is minimal to moderate in auditory toxicity, consider a trial use to determine if a patient with hearing loss can benefit from their use
Psychotic symptoms	**Cs** **H** Fq Eto/Pto	• Stop suspected agent for a short period of time (1–4 weeks) while psychotic symptoms are brought under control • Initiate antipsychotic therapy • Lower dose of suspected agent if this can be done without compromising regimen • Discontinue suspected agent if this can be done without compromising regimen • Some patients will need to continue antipsychotic treatment throughout MDR-TB treatment • Previous history of psychiatric disease is not a contraindication to the use of agents listed here but may increase the likelihood of psychotic symptoms developing during treatment • Psychotic symptoms are generally reversible upon completion of MDR-TB treatment or cessation of the offending agent
Depression	**Cs** Fq Eto/Pto H	• Offer group or individual counseling • Initiate antidepressant therapy • Lower dose of suspected agent if this can be done without compromising regimen • Discontinue suspected agent if this can be done without compromising regimen • Socioeconomic conditions and chronic illness should not be underestimated as contributing factors to depression • Depressive symptoms may fluctuate during therapy and may improve as illness is successfully treated • History of previous depression is not a contraindication to the use of the agents listed but may increase the likelihood of depression developing during treatment.

(Contd.)

(Contd.)

Adverse effect	Suspected agent	Suggested management strategies
Hypothyroidism	**PAS** **Eto/Pto**	• Initiate thyroxine therapy • Completely reversible upon discontinuation of PAS or ethionamide/prothionamide • The combination of ethionamide/prothionamide with PAS is more frequently associated with hypothyroidism than the individual use of each drug
Nausea and vomiting	**Eto/Pto** **PAS** H E Z Bdq Dlm	• Assess for dehydration; initiate rehydration if indicated • Initiate antiemetic therapy • Lower dose of suspected agent if this can be done without compromising regimen • Discontinue suspected agent if this can be done without compromising regimen rarely necessary • Nausea and vomiting universal in early weeks of therapy and usually abate with time on treatment and adjunctive therapy • Electrolytes should be monitored if vomiting is severe • Reversible upon discontinuation of suspected agent • Severe abdominal distress and acute abdomen have been reported with the use of clofazimine. Although these reports are rare, if this effect occurs, clofazimine should be suspended
Gastritis	**PAS** **Eto/Pto** Bdq Dlm	• H2-blockers, proton-pump inhibitors, or antacids • Stop suspected agent(s) for short periods of time (e.g. 1–7 days) • Lower dose of suspected agent, if this can be done without compromising regimen • Discontinue suspected agent if this can be done without compromising regimen • Severe gastritis, as manifested by hematemesis, melena or hematechezia, is rare • Dosing of antacids should be carefully timed so as to not interfere with the absorption of antituberculosis drugs (take 2 hours before or 3 hours after antituberculosis medications) • Reversible upon discontinuation of suspected agent(s)
Hepatitis	**Z** **H** **R** Eto/Pto PAS Fq	• Stop all therapy pending resolution of hepatitis • Eliminate other potential causes of hepatitis • Consider suspending most likely agent permanently • Reintroduce remaining drugs, one at a time while monitoring liver function • History of previous hepatitis should be carefully analyzed to determine most likely causative agent(s); these should be avoided in future regimens • Generally reversible upon discontinuation of suspected agent

(Contd.)

(Contd.)

Adverse effect	Suspected agent	Suggested management strategies
Renal toxicity	**S** **Km** **Am** **Cm**	• Discontinue suspected agent • Consider using capreomycin if an aminoglycoside had been the prior injectable in regimen • Consider dosing 2–3 times a week if drug is essential to the regimen and patient can tolerate (close monitoring of creatinine) • Adjust all antituberculosis medications according to the creatinine clearance • History of diabetes or renal disease is not a contraindication to the use of the agents listed here, although patients with these comorbidities may be at increased risk for developing renal failure • Renal impairment may be permanent
Electrolyte disturbances (hypokalemia and hypomagnesemia)	**Cm** **Km** **Am** S	• Check potassium • If potassium is low, also check magnesium (and calcium if hypocalcemia is suspected) • Replace electrolytes as needed • If severe hypokalemia is present, consider hospitalization • Amiloride 5–10 mg QD or spironolactone 25 mg QD may decrease potassium and magnesium wasting and is useful in refractory cases • Oral potassium replacements can cause significant nausea and vomiting. Oral magnesium may cause diarrhea
Optic neuritis	**E** Eto/Pto	• Stop E • Refer patient to an ophthalmologist • Usually reverses with cessation of E • Rare case reports of optic neuritis have been attributed to streptomycin
Arthralgias	**Z** Fq Bdq	• Initiate therapy with non-steroidal anti-inflammatory drugs • Lower dose of suspected agent if this can be done without compromising regimen • Discontinue suspected agent if this can be done without compromising regimen • Symptoms of arthralgia generally diminish over time, even without intervention • Uric acid levels may be elevated in patients on pyrazinamide. Allopurinol appears not to correct the uric acid levels in such cases

(H: isoniazid; R: rifampicin; E: ethambutol; Z: pyrazinamide; S: streptomycin; Km: kanamycin; Am: amikacin; Cm: capreomycin; Fq: fluoroquinolones; Eto: ethionamide; Pto: prothionamide; PAS: para-aminosalicylic acid; Cs: cycloserine; Cfz: clofazimine; Lzd: linezolid; Clr: Clarithromycin; Bdq: Bedaquiline; Dlm: delamanid)
Drugs that the strongly associated with adverse effects shown in bold.

CONCLUSION

The initial evaluation, timely and intensive monitoring for, and management of, adverse effects caused by second-line drugs are essential components of DR-TB control programs. Poor management of adverse effects increases the risk of default or irregular adherence to treatment, and may result in death or permanent morbidity. The physicians should be familiar with the common adverse effects of MDR-TB therapy. Patients experiencing adverse effects should be referred to specialists who have experience in treating the adverse effects. It is rarely necessary to suspend antituberculosis drugs completely. Ancillary drugs for the management of adverse effects should be available.

FURTHER READINGS

1. Companion Handbook to the WHO guidelines for the programmatic management of drug resistant tuberculosis. WHO/HTM/TB/2014.11.
2. Furin JJ, Mitnick CD, Shin SS, Bayona J, Becerra MC, Singler JM, et al. Occurrence of serious adverse effects in patients receiving community-based therapy for multidrug-resistant tuberculosis. International Journal of Tuberculosis and Lung Disease. 2001;5:648-55.
3. Guidelines for programmatic management of drug resistant tuberculosis. WHO, 2011. WHO/HTM/TB/2011.6
4. Guidelines for the programmatic management of drug-resistant tuberculosis: emergency update 2008. Geneva, World Health Organization, 2008 (WHO/HTM/TB/ 2008.402)
5. Nahid P, et al. ATS/CDC/IDSA Clinical Practice Guidelines: Treatment of drug-susceptible tuberculosis. Clin Infec Dis. 2016:1-50.
6. Nathanson E, Gupta R, Huamani P, Leimane V, Pasechnikov AD, Tupasi TE, et al. Adverse events in the treatment of multidrug-resistant tuberculosis: results from the DOTS-Plus initiative. International Journal of Tuberculosis and Lung Disease. 2004;8:1382-4.
7. Shin S, Furin J, Alcantara F, et al. Hypokalaemia among patients receiving treatment for multidrug-resistant tuberculosis. Chest. 2004;125:974-80.

CHAPTER

Antitubercular and Antiretroviral Drugs Interactions

Worldwide, tuberculosis (TB) is one of the most important infectious diseases in subjects with human immunodeficiency virus (HIV) infection. Rifamycin based antituberculosis therapy can cure HIV-related TB and, where available, the introduction of highly active antiretroviral therapy (HAART) has markedly reduced the incidence of acquired immunodeficiency syndromes (AIDS) and death. Although effective therapy is available for both conditions, there are major problems in the concurrent treatment of HIV and TB coinfection.

ANTIRETROVIRAL THERAPY FOR THE TREATMENT OF HIV INFECTION

Rapid progress in developing antiretroviral therapy (ART) led in 1996 the introduction of HAART. HAART is a combination of at least three antiretroviral (ARV) drugs. HAART is the global standard of care in the treatment of HIV infection. Although not a cure for HIV infection, HAART usually results in near-complete suppression of HIV replication. Treatment has to be lifelong. ART results in dramatic reductions in morbidity and mortality in HIV-infected people. There are several requirements for successful use of ART. These include considerable efforts to maintain adherence to lifelong treatment and to monitor response to treatment, drug toxicities and drug interactions.

Antiretroviral Drugs (ARV)

ARV drugs belong to following classes:

1. Reverse transcriptase inhibitors (RTIs),
2. Protease inhibitors (Pis),
3. Fusion or entry inhibitors and
4. Integrase Inhibitors.
5. CCR5 antagonist or entry inhibitors

RTIs are further divided into three groups:

i. Nucleoside reverse transcriptase inhibitors (NsRTIs);
ii. Non-nucleoside reverse transcriptase inhibitors (NNRTIs) and
iii. Nucleotide reverse transcriptase inhibitors (NtRTIs).

Nucleoside Reverse Transcriptase Inhibitors (NsRTIs)

NsRTI inhibit reverse transcription by being incorporated into the newly synthesized viral DNA and preventing its further elongation. Drugs available with their toxicities from this group are shown in Table 18.1.

TABLE 18.1: Nucleoside reverse transcriptase inhibitors (NsRTIs) with their toxicites.

Drugs	Abbreviation	Toxicity	Food Restriction
Zidovudine	AZT, ZDV	Anemia, granulocytopenia, myopathy, lactic acidosis, hepatomegaly with steatosis, headache and nausea	Taken with or without food
Didanosine	ddl	Pancreatitis, peripheral neuropathy, abnormalities in liver function tests, lactic acidosis, hepatomegaly with steatosis	Taken on an empty stomach 30 minutes before, or 2 hours after a meal
Stavudine	d4T	Peripheral neuropathy, pancreatitis, lactic acidosis, hepatomegaly with steatosis, ascending neuromuscular weakness and lipodystrophy	Taken with or without food
Lamivudine	3TC	Headache and dry mouth	Taken with or without food
Zalcitabine	ddC	Peripheral neuropathy, pancreatitis, lactic acidosis, hepatomegaly with steatosis and oral ulcers	Taken with or without food
Emtricitabine	FTC	Headache, nausea, insomnia, hypertrophy of palms and soles	Taken with or without food
Abacavir	ABC	Hypersensitivity reaction (can be fatal); fever, rash, nausea, vomiting, malaise or fatigue, and loss of appetite	Taken with or without food

Nucleotide Reverse Transcriptase Inhibitors (NtRTIs)

Mechanism of action is similar to NsRTIs, it undergoes diester hydrolysis to form the nucleoside monophosphate tenofovir. Drugs available with their toxicities from this group are shown in Table 18.2.

TABLE 18.2: Nucleotide reverse transcriptase inhibitors (NtRTIs) with toxicity.

Drug	Abbreviation	Toxicity	Food restriction
Tenofovir	TDF	Potential for renal toxicity	Taken with or without food

Non-nucleoside Reverse Transcriptase Inhibitors (NNRTIs)

NNRTIs inhibit reverse transcriptase directly by binding to the enzyme and interfering with its function. Drugs available with their toxicities from this group are shown in Table 18.3.

TABLE 18.3: Non-nucleoside reverse transcriptase inhibitors (NNRTIs) with their toxicites.

Drugs	Abbreviation	Toxicity	Food restriction
Delavirdine	DLV	Skin rash, abnormalities in liver function tests	Taken with or without food
Efavirenz	EFV	Rash, dysphoria, elevated liver function tests, drowsiness, abnormal dreams, depression	Taken on empty stomach
Nevirapine	NVP	Skin rash, hepatotoxicity	Taken with or without food
Etravirine	ETR	Elevation in liver function tests	Taken following a meal

Protease Inhibitors (PIs)

PIs target viral assembly by inhibiting the activity of protease, an enzyme used by HIV to cleave nascent proteins for final assembly of new virions. Drugs available with their toxicities from this group are shown in Table 18.4.

TABLE 18.4: Protease Inhibitors (PIs) with their toxicites.

Drugs	Abbreviation	Toxicity	Food restriction
Amprenavir	APV	Nausea, vomiting, diarrhea, rash, oral paresthesias, elevated liver function tests, hyperglycemia, fat redistribution, lipid abnormalities	Taken with or without food; avoid high fat meals
Fosamprenavir	FOS-APV	Vomiting, elevated liver function tests, hyperglycemia, fat redistribution	Taken with or without food
Atazanavir	ATV	Hyperbilirubinemia,PR prolongation, nausea, vomiting, hyperglycemia, fat maldistribution	Taken with food
Darunavir	DRV	Diarrhea nausea, headache	Taken with food
Indinavir	IDV	Nephrolithiasis, hypergly-cemia, fat redistribution, lipid abnormalities, indirect hyperbilirubinemia	Taken on an empty stomach 60 minutes before, or 2 hours after a meal. Avoid taking within an hour of taking didanosine
Lopinavir/ Ritonavir	LPV/RTV	Diarrhea, hyperglycemia, fat redistribution, lipid abnormalities	
Nelfinavir	NFV	Diarrhea, loose stools, hyperglycemia, fat redistribution, lipid abnormalities	Taken with food

(Contd.)

(Contd.)

Drugs	Abbreviation	Toxicity	Food restriction
Ritonavir	RTV	Nausea, abdominal pain, hyperglycemia, fat redistribution, lipid abnormalities, may alter levels of many other drugs, including saquinavir	Taken with food
Saquinavir	SQV	Diarrhea, nausea, headaches, hyperglycemia, fat redistribution, lipid abnormalities	Taken within two hours of food
Tipranavir	TPV	Nausea, vomiting, diarrhea, elevation in liver function tests, increased total cholesterol and triglyceride, rash and intracranial hemorrhages	Taken with or without food

Fusion Inhibitors

Fusion inhibitors block the HIV envelope from merging with the host CD4 cell membrane (fusion). This prevents HIV from entering the CD4 cell. Drugs available with their toxicities from this group are shown in Table 18.5.

TABLE 18.5: Fusion inhibitors with their toxicities

Drug	Abbreviation	Toxicity	Food restriction
Enfuvirtide	T-20	Local injection reactions, hypersensitivity reactions, increased rate of bacterial pneumonia	Taken with or without food

Integrase Inhibitors

It inhibit the enzyme integrase, which is responsible for integration of viral DNA into the DNA of the infected cell. Drugs available with their toxicities from this group are shown in Table 18.6.

TABLE 18.6: Integrase inhibitors with toxicity.

Drugs	Abbreviation	Toxicity	Food restriction
Raltegravir	RAL	Nausea, diarrhea, elevation in amylases, dizziness, pruritus and rash	Taken with or without food
Elvitegravir	EVG	Diarrhea, allergic reactions, deranged liver function, IRIS	Taken with food
Dolutegravir	DTG	Allergic reactions, rash, liver problems, changes in body fat, IRIS, disturbed sleep, tiredness, headache	Taken with or without food

CCR5 Antagonist or Entry Inhibitors

CCR5 antagonists block the CCR5 coreceptor on the surface of certain immune cells, such as CD4 T lymphocytes (CD4 cells). This prevents HIV from entering the cell. Drugs available with their toxicities from this group are shown in Table 18.7.

TABLE 18.7: CCR5 antagonists with toxicity.

Drug	Abbreviation	Toxicity	Food restriction
Maraviroc	MVC	Diarrhea, nausea, fatigueness, cough, headache, joint pain, muscle pain, hepatitis	Must be prepared from a powder and injected into thigh, arm or abdomen

Pharmacokinetic Issues in the Treatment of HIV-related Tuberculosis

Two pharmacokinetic issues complicate the treatment of HIV-related tuberculosis: The possibility of malabsorption of antituberculosis drugs, and the complex drug-drug interactions. There are conflicting data on whether patients with HIV-related tuberculosis are more prone to malabsorption of antituberculosis drugs than are HIV-uninfected patients. It appears that serum drug concentrations, particularly of rifampin, are somewhat lower in tuberculosis patients with HIV infection and very low CD4 cell count.

Interaction between Antiretroviral and Antitubercular Drugs

Treatment of TB in the presence of HIV infection is complicated by drug-drug interactions between the rifamycin class of antimycobacterial drugs (rifampin, rifabutin and rifapentine), and the PI and the NNRTI classes of drugs used to treat HIV infection. Both PIs and NNRTIs are metabolized by hepatic CYP3A, especifically the CYP3A4 isozyme. Rifamycins are inducers of the CYP3A family of enzymes, which includes the CYP3A4 isozyme. This will adversely affect the ability of the antiretroviral regimen to adequately suppress the virus, which is the goal of antiretroviral treatment regimen.

Rifamycins and Nucleoside/Nucleotide Analogues

Rifamycins are inducers of the CYP3A system but rifampin is not metabolized by this system. Of the three available rifamycins, rifampin is the most potent inducer of CYP3A and rifabutin is the least potent, with rifapentine falling somewhere in between. Rifapentine should not be used for the treatment of TB in HIV-infected individuals because of the increased rate of acquired rifamycin resistance. Rifabutin has been used extensively in the developed world as a substitute for rifampin in the treatment of active TB, outcomes are similar with rifampin or rifabutin. Rifabutin is metabolized by the CYP3A system and there is significant interactions when rifabutin is coadministred with PIs and NNRTIs. Rifabutin dosing has to be adjusted according to the choice of the coadministered antiretroviral.

Rifamycins and Protease Inhibitor

Protease inhibitors (PIs) and the rifamycins have opposite effects on CYP3A family of enzymes in the liver. This causes the following types of drug-drug interactions when PIs are taken together with rifamycins: PI serum concentrations and overall bioavailability may decrease to subtherapeutic levels because rifamycins accelerate the metabolism of PIs by inducing the CYP3 enzymes. Rifampin levels are not affected since it is not metabolized by the CYP3A and rifabutin bioavailability may increase to toxic levels because PIs decrease its metabolism. Rifampicin causes a 75–95% reduction in serum concentrations of PI other than ritonavir. Such reductions lead to loss of antiretroviral activity of PI-containing regimens and consequently can result in the emergence of resistance to one or more of the other drugs in the HAART regimen. Currently, most patients are given combinations of PI, which includes low dose ritonavir [usually 100 mg per dose] in order to take advantage of its enzyme inhibiting properties. In effect ritonavir boosts the concentrations of the other PI allowing easier and more tolerable dosing. Rifabutin can be used with single (unboosted) PI except saquinavir. However, because of the balance between rifabutin induction and protease inhibition of CYP3A4, when this combination is used a modification in the dose of the PI may be required and the dose of rifabutin should be decreased by half to 150 mg.

Rifamycins and Non-nucleoside Reverse Transcriptase Inhibitors

The NNRTIs are all metabolized by the hepatic CYP3A. Therefore, NNRTI levels are adversely affected by the rifamycins. The effect of NNRTIs on the CYP3A is less uniform; delavirdine inhibits the CYP3A, whereas nevirapine and efavirenz induce the CYP3A. Delavirdine should not be used with either rifampin or rifabutin because both rifamycins greatly diminish the levels of delavirdine. Rifampin modestly decreases the efavirenz activity. Therefore, it is probably safe to use rifampin concomitantly with efavirenz at a slightly higher dose (800 mg of efavirenz instead of the usual 600 mg). Efavirenz effectiveness is not significantly affected by rifabutin, but efavirenz does decrease rifabutin bioavailability. Therefore, the rifabutin dosage must be increased (from the usual dosage of 300 mg to a daily dose of 450–600 mg) when it is given with efavirenz. Bioavailability of nevirapine is reduced by rifampin. Rifabutin decreases bioavailabilty of nevirapine and nevirapine also slightly decreases rifabutin bioavailability. Therefore, nevirapine can be used with rifabutin, both at their usual doses.

Rifamycins and Nucleoside Reverse Transcriptase Inhibitors (NRTIs)

There is a slight decrease in the level of zidovudine and probably abacavir when coadministered with rifampin. The other NRTIs do not interact significantly with rifamycins. Rifamycins can therefore be included in the anti-TB regimen if a PI- or NNRTI-sparing antiretroviral regimen is chosen. The fusion inhibitor enfuvirtide, is not known to be a substrate for the CYP450 enzymes or to have any effect on the levels of these enzymes and can be used with all anti-TB drugs.

Isoniazid and Antiretroviral Drug Interactions

Pharmacokinetic or clinical interactions between isoniazid and antiretroviral agents have not been extensively studied. In vitro studies have shown that isoniazid, at clinically relevant concentrations, is a reversible inhibitor of CYP3A4 and CYP2C19, and that it mechanistically inactivates CYP1A2, CYP2A6, CYP2C19 and CYP3A4 in human liver microsomes. Isoniazid, coadministered with drugs such as PI and NNRTI, which are metabolized by these isoforms, may result in significant drug-drug interactions. These interactions might be significant when isoniazid is given alone to treat latent TB infection in an HIV coinfected patient who is receiving PI or NNRTI.

Drug–drug Interactions in the Treatment of HIV and Drug Resistant-TB (DR-TB)

Currently, little is known about drug–drug interactions between second-line antituberculosis agents and antiretroviral therapy. Buffered didanosine contains an aluminium/magnesium-based antacid and, if given jointly with fluoroquinolones, may result in decreased fluoroquinolone absorption; it should be avoided, but if it is necessary it should be given six hours before or two hours after fluoroquinolone administration. The enteric coated formulation of didanosine can be used concomitantly without this precaution. Ethionamide/protionamide is thought to be metabolized by the CYP450 system, although it is not known which of the CYP enzymes are responsible. Whether doses of ethionamide/protionamide and/or certain antiretroviral drugs should be modified during the concomitant treatment of DR-TB and HIV is completely unknown. Clarithromycin is a substrate and inhibitor of CYP3A and has multiple drug interactions with protease inhibitors and NNRTIs. If possible, the use of clarithromycin should be avoided in patients coinfected with DR-TB and HIV because of its weak efficacy against DR-TB and multiple drug interactions and added adverse event. Bedaquiline is metabolized by the CYP3A4 and has multiple drug interactions with protease inhibitors and non-nucleoside reverse-transcriptase inhibitors (NNRTIs). CYP3A4 is the metabolizer of delamanid. Many drugs can either induce or inhibit the CYP3A4 system, resulting in drug–drug interactions.

CONCLUSION

With non-rifamycin containing regimens, drug-drug interactions might be fewer but a non-rifamycin regimen is inferior to a rifampicin-based regimen for the treatment of HIV-related tuberculosis. These should be only contemplated in patients with serious toxicity to rifamycins, where desensitization/reintroduction has failed, or in those with rifamycin-resistant isolates.The various options to reduce drug-drug interactions are: (i) to postpone antiretroviral therapy, (ii) to use no PI or NNRTI containing antiretroviral combinations, (iii) to use certain PI/ and/or NNRTIs with modification in doses, (iv) Efavirenz (EFZ) or saquinavir with ritonavir, without the need to adjust the doses, (v) to use non rifamycin regimens, e.g. 2 SHEZ + 10 HE.

FURTHER READINGS

1. CDC. Managing Drug Interactions in the Treatment of HIV-Related Tuberculosis [online]. 2013. Available from URL: http://www.cdc.gov/tb/TB_HIV_Drugs/default.htm
2. Centers for Disease Control and Prevention (CDC). Managing drug interactions in the treatment of HIV-related tuberculosis [online]. 2007 (available at http://www.cdc. Gov/tb/TB_ HIV_ Drugs/default.htm.
3. Consolidated guidelines on the use of antiretroviral drugs for treating and preventing HIV infection: recommendations for a public health approach – 2nd edition. WHO; 2016.
4. Corbett EL, Watt CJ, Walker N, et al. The growing burden of tuberculosis: global trends and interactions with the HIV epidemic. Arch Intern Med. 2003;163:1009-21.
5. Desta Z, Soukhova NV, Flockhart DA. Inhibition of cytochrome P450 (CYP450) by isoniazid: potent inhibition of CYP2C19 and CYP3A. Antimicrob Agents Chemother. 2001;45:382-92.
6. Sahai J, Gallicano K, Swick L, Tailor S, Garber G, Seguin I, et al. Reduced plasma concentrations of antituberculous drugs in patients with HIV infection. Ann Intern Med. 1997;127:289-93.
7. TB/HIV Clinical manual. second edition. WHO/HTM/TB/2004.329.
8. UNIADS/WHO. AIDS epidemic update: December 2003. UNAIDS/WHO 2003. http://www.unaids.org/wad/2003/epiupdate2003.

CHAPTER

Adverse Drug Reactions of Antiretroviral Therapy and Antituberculosis Therapy

Potential overlying and additive toxicities of antiretroviral therapy and antituberculosis therapy with their management is tabulated in Table 19.1. Drugs that are more strongly associated with adverse effects appear in bold.

TABLE 19.1: Potential overlying and additive toxicities of antiretroviral therapy and antituberculosis therapy.

Toxicity	Antiretroviral agent	Antituberculosis agent	Comments
Peripheral neuropathy	D4T (stavudine) ddl (didanosine), ddC (zalcitabine)	Lzd (linezolid) Cs (cycloserine) H (isoniazid) Aminoglycosides Eto (ethionamide) Pto (prothionamide) E (ethambutol)	• Avoid use of D4T, ddI and ddC in combination with Cs or Lzd because of increased peripheral neuropathy • If these agents are to be used and peripheral neuropathy develops, replace the ARV agent with a less neurotoxic agent
Central nervous system toxicity	Efavirenz (EFV)	Cs (cycloserine) H (isoniazid) Eto (ethionamide) Pto (prothionamide) Fluoroquinolones	• Efavirenz has a high rate of CNS adverse effects (confusion, impaired concentration, depersonalization, abnormal dreams, insomnia and dizziness) in the first 2–3 weeks, which typically resolve on their own. If these effects do not resolve on their own, consider substitution of the agent
Depression	Efavirenz (EFV)	Cs(cycloserine), Fluoroquinolones H (isoniazid) Eto (ethionamide) Pto (prothionamide)	• Severe depression can be seen in 2.4% of patients receiving EFV. Consider substituting for EFV if severe depression develops

(Contd.)

(Contd.)

Toxicity	Antiretroviral agent	Antituberculosis agent	Comments
Headache	AZT (zidovudine), EFV (efavirenz)	Cs (cycloserine) Bdq (bedaquiline)	• Rule out more serious causes of headache such as bacterial meningitis, cryptococcal meningitis, CNS toxoplasmosis • Use of analgesics (ibuprofen, paracetamol) and good hydration may help • Headache secondary to AZT, EFV and Cs is usually self-limited
Nausea and vomiting	RTV (ritonavir), D4T (stavudine) NVP (nevirapine)	Eto (Ethionamide) Pto (prothionamide) PAS (para-amino salicylic acid) H (isoniazid) Bdq (bedaquiline) Dlm (delamanid) E (ethambutol) Z (pyrazimamide)	• Nausea and vomiting are common adverse effects and can be managed • Persistent vomiting and abdominal pain may be a result of developing lactic acidosis and/or hepatitis secondary to medications
Abdominal pain	All ART treatment has been associated with abdominal pain	Cfz Eto/Pto PAS	• Abdominal pain is a common adverse effect and often benign; however, abdominal pain may be an early symptom of severe adverse effects such as pancreatitis, hepatitis or lactic acidosis
Pancreatitis	D4T (stavudine) ddI (didanosine) ddC (zalcitabine)	Lzd (linezolid)	• Avoid use of these agents together. If an agent causes pancreatitis suspend it and do not use any of the pancreatitis producing anti-HIV medications (D4T, ddI, or ddC) in the future • Also consider gallstones or alcohol as a potential cause of pancreatitis
Diarrhea	All protease inhibitors, ddI (didanosine)	Eto (ethionamide)/ Pto (prothiona-mide), PAS (para-amino-salicylic acid). Flour-oquinolones	• Diarrhea is a common adverse effect • Also consider opportunistic infections as a cause of diarrhea, or clostridium difficile (a cause of pseudomembranous colitis)

(Contd.)

(Contd.)

Toxicity	Antiretroviral agent	Antituberculosis agent	Comments
Hepatotoxicity	NVP (nevirapine) EFV (efavirenz), All protease inhibitors all NRTIs	H (isoniazid) R (rifampicin) E (ethambutol) Z (pyrazinamide) Bdq (bedaquiline) PAS (para-amino salicylic acid) Eto (ethionamide) Pto (prothionamide) Fluoroquinolones	• Also consider TMP/SMX as a cause of hepatotoxicity if the patient is receiving this medication • Also rule out viral etiologies as cause of hepatitis (Hepatitis A, B, C, and CMV)
Skin rash	ABC (abacavir) NVP (nevirapine), EFV (efavirenz) D4T (stavudine)	H (isoniazid) R (rifampicin) Z (pyrazinamide) PAS (para-amino salicylic acid) Fluoroquinolones	• Do not re-challenge with ABC (can result in life-threatening anaphylaxis) • Do not re-challenge with an agent that caused Stevens-Johnson syndrome • Also consider TMP/SMX as a cause of skin rash if the patient is receiving this medication • Thioacetazone is contraindicated in HIV because of life-threatening rash
Lactic acidosis	D4T (stavudine) ddI (didanosine), AZT (zidovudine) 3TC (lamivudine)	Lzd (linezolid)	• If an agent causes lactic acidosis, replace it with an agent less likely to cause lactic acidosis
Renal toxicity	TDF(tenofovir)	Aminoglycosides cm (capreomycin)	• TDF may cause renal injury with the characteristic features of Fanconi syndrome, hypophosphatemia, hypouricemia, proteinuria, normoglycemic glycosuria and, in some cases, acute renal failure • Use TDF with caution in patients receiving aminoglycosides or Cm • Frequent creatinine and electrolyte monitoring every 1 to 3 weeks is recommended
Nephrolithiasis	IDV (indinavir)	None	• No overlapping toxicities regarding nephrolithiasis have been documented between ART and antituberculosis medications

(Contd.)

(Contd.)

Toxicity	Antiretroviral agent	Antituberculosis agent	Comments
			• Adequate hydration prevents nephrolithiasis in patients taking IDV • If nephrolithiasis develops while on IDV, substitute with another protease inhibitor if possible
Electrolyte disturbances	TDF (tenofovir)	Cm (capreomycin) Aminoglycosides	• Diarrhea and/or vomiting can contribute to electrolyte disturbances • Even without the concurrent use of TDF, HIV-infected patients have an increased risk of both renal toxicity and electrolyte disturbances secondary to aminoglycosides and Cm
Bone marrow suppression	AZT (zidovudine)	Lzd (linezolid), R (rifampicin) Rfb (rifabutin) H (isoniazid)	• Monitor blood counts regularly. Replace AZT if bone marrow suppression develops. Consider suspension of Lzd • Also consider TMP/SMX as a cause if the patient is receiving this medication • Consider adding folinic acid supplements, especially if receiving TMP/SMX
Optic neuritis	ddI (didanosine)	E (Ethambutol), Eto (ethionamide) Pto (prothionamide)	• Suspend agent responsible for optic neuritis permanently and replace with an agent that does not cause optic neuritis
Hyperlipidemia	Protease-inhibitors EFV (efavirenz)	None	• No overlapping toxicities regarding hyperlipidemia have been documented between ART and antituberculosis medications
Lipodystrophy	NRTIs (especially D4T (stavudine) and ddI (didanosine)	None	• No overlapping toxicities regarding lipodystrophy have been documented between ART and antituberculosis medications

(Contd.)

(Contd.)

Toxicity	Antiretroviral agent	Antituberculosis agent	Comments
Dysglycemia (disturbed blood sugar regulation)	Protease inhibitors	Gfx (gatifloxicin) Eto (ethionamide) Pto (prothionamide)	• Protease inhibitors tend to cause insulin resistance and hyperglycemia • Eto/Pto tend to make insulin control in diabetics more difficult, and can result in hypoglycemia and poor glucose regulation
Hypothyroidism	D4T (stavudine)	Eto (ethionamide) Pto (prothionamide) PAS (para-amino-salicylic acid)	• There is potential for overlying toxicity, but evidence is mixed • Several studies show subclinical hypothyroidism associated with HAART, particularly stavudine • PAS and Eto/Pto, especially in combination can commonly cause hypothyroidism
Arthralgia	Indinavir, other protease inhibitors	Z (pyrazinamide), Bdq (bedaquiline)	• Protease inhibitors can cause arthralgia and there have been case reports of more severe rheumatologic pathology • Arthralgias are very common with Z and has been reported as one of the most frequent adverse effects (>10%) in controlled clinical trials with Bdq
QT Prolongation	ART has been associated with QTc prolongation	Bdq (bedaquiline), Dlm (delamanid), Mfx (moxifloxacin), Gfx (gatifloxicin), Cfz (clofazamine), Lfx (levofloxacin), Ofx (ofloxacin)	• ARV therapy does appear to confer a significant increased risk of QTc prolongation in HIV-positive patients but data is sparse • The additive effects of combining ART with the known second-line anti-TB drugs in respect to QTc prolongation is not known

FURTHER READINGS

1. Centers for Disease Control and Prevention (CDC). Managing drug interactions in the treatment of HIV-related tuberculosis. 2007 (available at http :// www .cdc. Gov /tb/ TB_ HIV_ Drugs/default.htm.

2. Companion Handbook to the WHO guidelines for the programmatic management of drug resistant tuberculosis. WHO/HTM/TB/2014.11.
3. Consolidated guidelines on the use of antiretroviral drugs for treating and preventing HIV infection: recommendations for a public health approach – 2nd edition. WHO; 2016.
4. Guidelines for programmatic management of drug resistant tuberculosis. WHO, 2011. WHO/HTM/TB/2011.6
5. TB/HIV Clinical manual. second edition. WHO/HTM/TB/2004.329.
6. World Health Organisation 2012. WHO policy on collaborative TB/HIV activities guidelines for national programmes and other stakeholders. WHO/HTM/TB/2012;WHO/HIV/2012.1.
7. World Health Organization. Guidance for National Tuberculosis and HIV Programmes on the management of tuberculosis in HIV-infected children: recommendations for a public health approach. Geneva: World Health Organization; 2010.

CHAPTER

Epidemiology of Adverse Drug Reactions in New Patients of Tuberculosis

India features among the 22 high tuberculosis (TB) burden countries and has accounted for an estimated one-quarter (26%) of all TB cases worldwide. Treatment regimen with multiple first-line antitubercular agents (isoniazid, rifampicin, pyrazinamide, ethambutol, streptomycin) remains the cornerstone of treatment of tuberculosis. Good bacteriological diagnosis and compliance on treatment are the two main pillars of successful treatment of pulmonary tuberculosis. Adverse reactions to these agents are common and cause significant morbidity and even sometimes mortality if not detected early. The World Health Organization (WHO) has defined adverse drug reactions (ADRs) as "A response to a drug which is noxious and unintended, and which occurs at doses normally used in human for the prophylaxis, diagnosis, or therapy of disease, or for the modification of physiological function." Timing, the pattern of illness, the results of investigations, and re-challenge will help attribute causality to a suspected ADR. Various factors such as the dose and time of day at which the medication is administered, patient age, nutritional status, the presence of pre-existing diseases or dysfunctions like impaired liver function, impaired kidney function, HIV coinfection, and alcoholism may be related to adverse reactions to antituberculosis drugs. This calls for continued surveillance of ADRs, especially in public health programs that treat large number of patients, especially in disease like tuberculosis where early recognition and appropriate management of ADRs might determine adherence and therefore treatment success.

PREVALENCE OF ADRS WITH FIRST-LINE ANTITUBERCULAR DRUGS-GLOBAL SCENARIO

The data on global prevalence of ADRs with first-line antitubercular drugs are scarce. The prevalence of ADRs observed in various studies conducted worldwide ranged from 8% to 85% as mentioned in Table 20.1. This table has focused primarily on those studies that have adopted programmatic treatment approach known as Directly Observed Treatment and Short course chemotherapy (DOTS). The reasons for variation in the prevalence of ADRs across various studies might be related to several possible factors such as: differences in definitions of ADRs terminologies as adopted by clinicians, whether the ADRs were reported subjectively by patient or objectively by clinician on the basis of clinical evidence and monitoring with serial laboratory investigations, the differences in existing comorbid illnesses such as diabetes, hypertension, or hypothyroidism, and other co-variates including HIV coinfection and variations in the use of specific anti-tubercular drugs including dosage and also pharmacological interactions with other group of drugs particularly antiretroviral therapy. A study conducted in Nigeria observed that around 14% and 13% incidence of ADRs at 6 months and 8 months, among patients receiving DOTS respectively. In another study conducted by the Hong-Kong Chest Services, ADRs were observed in 21% of patients receiving intermittent therapy. Brazilian National Ministry of Health reported the incidence of minor or mild ADRs in patients treated with the former first-line ATT to range from 5% to 20%. It was also observed that major or severe ADRs were less common (occurring in approximately 2% of the cases, reaching 8% in specialized clinics) and led to the discontinuation or alteration of the treatment. However, another study from a teaching hospital in Brazil reported that 41.1% of the patients presented with minor and 12.8% presented with major ADRs. In a study from Singapore, frequency of ADRs was observed to be 28.7% whereas it was observed to be 29.27% from another study conducted at Hong Kong. However, studies have revealed that there are no differential rates of ADRs among patients having intermittent and daily intake of antituberculosis drugs. It was also observed that ADRs were more prevalent in intensive phase than continuation phase.

PREVALENCE OF ADRS WITH FIRST-LINE ANTITUBERCULAR DRUGS—INDIA

The Revised National Tuberculosis Control Program (RNTCP) has adopted the principles of DOTS and has been treating patients of pulmonary tuberculosis throughout the country since 1998. It has achieved global benchmark of treatment success consecutively for the last five years. The overall prevalence of ADRs with first-line antituberculosis drugs is estimated to vary from 2.3% to 17% in various Indian studies. A study conducted by Mehrotra et al. observed that the prevalence of ADRs in the initial intensive phase was 17.39%. Another study conducted at a tertiary institute in Calcutta observed that the overall toxicity was found in 35% cases in the daily regimen group, whereas it was found to be 27.9% in the intermittent regimen group. Data regarding prevalence of ADRs are still scarce and further surveys are required from different geographical areas of India in near future.

TABLE 20.1: Characteristics of important studies showing frequency of adverse drug reactions due to first-line antituberculosis drugs.

Study year	Location	Sample size	Study period	Type of regimen	Duration of treatment (months)	Number of drugs in regimens	Incidence of ADRs (%)	Profile of ADRs
Dosumu (2002)	Nigeria	Group 1–500 Group 2–50	Jan 1996–Dec 1997	DOTS (CAT 1)	6–8	5	Group 1–13 Group 2–14	Group 1 – Arthralgia (4%), pruritus (2%), fever (2%), systemic flu like syndrome (2%), gastroenteritis-nausea and vomiting (1.6%), jaundice (1%), maculopapular rash (0.4%) Group 2 – Arthralgia (4%), pruritus (2%), fever (2%), systemic flu like syndrome (4%), jaundice (2%)
Yee (2003)	Canada	430	1990–1999	Supervised/DOTS	6–8	4	10.70	Rash/Drug fever (4.88%), hepatitis (2.79%), severe gastrointestinal upset (2.56%), visual toxicity (0.23%), arthralgia (0.23%)
Dhingra (2004)	India	1195	Jan 2002–Jun 2003	DOTS	6–9	5	8.37	Nausea and vomiting (53%), general aches and pain (35%), giddiness (27%), skin rash and itching (17%), arthralgia (11%), hepatotoxicity (1%)
Gülbay (2006)	Turkey	1149	1984–2001	DOTS	9	4–5	9.00	Hepatotoxicity – Functional liver disturbance (4.9%), hepatotoxicity (2.4%), severe hepatotoxicity (0.8%), hyperuricemia (including arthralgia) – (2.6%), ototoxicity (1.7%), psychiatric changes (0.7%), cutaneous reactions (0.6%), flu-like syndrome (0.3%), gluteal abscess (0.2%), fever (0.2%), peripheral neuropathy (0.1%), changes in visual acuity (0.1%), hemolytic reaction (0.1%), change in glucose tolerance (0.1%)
Gholami (2006)	Iran	83	Jul 2001–Jul 2002	DOTS	6	4	53.01	Hepatitis (25.9%), Constipation (17.3%), increased liver transaminases (11.2%), hyperglycemia (8.7%), headache (8.7%), peripheral neuropathy (6.2%), dysuria (4.9%), rash (4.9%), diarrhea (3.7%), increased uric acid (3.7%), vision abnormality (2.4%), prolonged prothrombin time (2.4%)

Contd...

Contd...

Study year	Location	Sample size	Study period	Type of regimen	Duration of treatment (months)	Number of drugs in regimens	Incidence of ADRs (%)	Profile of ADRs
Taher (2006)	India	1490	Dec 2002–Aug 2005	DOTS	6–9	5	29.00	Nausea and vomiting (11%), transient gastritis (9%), elevated serum aspartate aminotransferase or alanine aminotransferase (>50 iu/l) (3%), elevated serum alkaline
Kishore (2008)	Nepal	326	Jan 2001–Dec 2006	DOTS	6–9	5	12.27	Elevated hepatic enzymes/Hepatitis (57.14%), gastritis (9.52%), arthralgia (9.52%), erythematous/macular rash (7.14%), interstitial nephritis/renal failure (4.76%), nausea/vomiting (4.76%), peripheral neuritis (2.38%), vestibular neuritis (2.38%), defective vision (2.38%)
Chhetri (2008)	Nepal	137	Jan 2005–Jun 2005	DOTS	6–9	5	54.74	Tingling and burning sensation in extremities (11.03%), joint pain (10.34%), bodyache (10.34%), epigastric burning (10.34%), generalized itching/rashes (10%), anorexia/nausea/vomiting (9.66%), vertigo/dizziness (6.21%), headache (4.83%), weakness (3.45%), tinnitus (2.41%), ataxia (1.72%), constipation (1.03%), diarrhea (1.03%), miscellaneous (7.93%)
Tak (2009)	India	94	Oct 2005–May 2006	DOTS	6–9	5	17.02	Gastritis (32.09%), hepatitis (9.52%), anorexia (4.76%), skin reactions (14.28%), peripheral neuropathy (4.76%), dizziness (4.76%), psychosis (4.76%), ototoxicity (4.76%), vertigo (4.76%), arthralgia (4.76%)

Contd...

Contd...

Study year	Location	Sample size	Study period	Type of regimen	Duration of treatment (months)	Number of drugs in regimens	Incidence of ADRs (%)	Profile of ADRs
Jeong (2009)	Korea	105	6 months	Supervised/ DOTS	6–8	5	57.00	Dermatologic (9%), GI trouble (8%), arthralgia (6%), visual change (6%), hepatotoxicity (4%), fatigue or malaise (6%), dizziness (4%), fever (1%)
Maciel (2010)	Brazil	79	2003–2006	Supervised/ DOTS	6	4	83.54	Joint pain (14.48%), skin edema or irritation (or both) (8.54%), memory loss (7.12%), acne (6.88%), itching (6.65%), epigastric or abdominal pain (or both) (5.46%), nausea or vomiting (or both) (4.98%), muscle pain (4.41%), headache (3.55%), painful limbs (3.55%), chest pain (2.74%), somnolence (2.69%), cough/sore throat/ presence of secretion (2.69%), pulmonary rhonchi or sounds (or both) (2.37%), weakness/ dyspnea (2.22%), eye irritation (2.22%), decreased visual acuity (2.22%), dysuria (1.67%), swelling of joints or bone (or both) (1.42%), hepatomegaly (1.42%), insomnia (1.42%), petechiae or bleeding (or both) (1.42%), alopecia (1.18%), myalgia (1.18%), loss of appetite (1.18%), dizziness (1.18%), adenopathy (0.94%) intolerance to light (0.94%), tremors (0.94%), anemia (0.47%), confusion or lack of attention (or both) (0.47%), fever (0.47%), lymph node enlargement (0.47%), depression (0.23%), sweats (0.23%)

Contd...

Contd...

Study year	Location	Sample size	Study period	Type of regimen	Duration of treatment (months)	Number of drugs in regimens	Incidence of ADRs (%)	Profile of ADRs
Gillani (2012)	Malaysia	653	Jan 2008–Jun 2010	Supervised/ DOTS	6–12	4	15.8	Skin reaction-itchiness, rashes (7.8%), gastrointestinal reactions-nausea, vomiting, GI upset (2.5%), Hepatotoxicity-hepatitis (2.6%), Central nervous system reactions-dizziness, headache (0.3%), skin along with gastrointestinal reactions (0.8%), skin along with central nervous system reactions (0.9%), gastrointestinal along with central nervous system reactions (0.6%), gastrointestinal along with skin reaction and muscle ache (0.2%), and skin reaction along with flu like syndrome (0.2%)
Lv (2013)	China	4304	Oct 2007–Jun 2008	DOTS	6–9	5	17.33	Liver dysfunction (6.34%), gastrointestinal disorders (3.74%), arthralgia (2.51%), allergic reactions (2.35%), nervous system disorders including ototoxicity (2.04%), hematologic system disorders (0.70%), renal impairment (0.07%), others (0.05%)
Sinha (2013)	India	102	Jul 2009–Dec 2010	DOTS	6–9	5	69.01	Anorexia (31.58%), vomiting (28.95%), nausea (21.05%), burning epigastrium (18.42%), generalized weakness (16.9%), liver dysfunction (15.49%), allergic skin reactions (8.45%), neurological (2.82%), fever (2.82%)
Qureshi (2013)	India	50	1.6 years	DOTS (CAT 1)	6	4	60.00	Nausea (56%), vomiting (30%), dyspepsia (24%), abdominal pain (20%), loss of taste (14%), diarrhea (4%), malaise (16%), jaundice (8%), skin rash (2%)

Contd...

Contd...

Study year	Location	Sample size	Study period	Type of regimen	Duration of treatment (months)	Number of drugs in regimens	Incidence of ADRs (%)	Profile of ADRs
Mandal (2013)	India	83 (Intermittent regimen-43) (Daily regimen-40)	Jan 2010–Dec 2011	DOTS (Intermittent and daily regimens)	6–9	5	Intermittent regimen – 25.58 Daily regimen – 35.00	Intermittent regimen – Gastrointestinal disturbance (9.30%), raised serum transaminase (6.98%), clinical jaundice (2.32%), vertigo (4.64%), itching & rash (2.32%), peripheral neuropathy (0.00%), arthralgia (0.00%) Daily regimen – Gastrointestinal disturbance (15.00%), raised serum transaminase (0.00%), clinical jaundice (7.5%), vertigo (0.00%), itching and rash (5.00%), peripheral neuropathy (2.50%), arthralgia (5.00%)
Dalal (2014)	India	150	Oct 2011–May 2013	DOTS	6–9	5	19.33	Gastrointestinal tolerance – Nausea/vomiting/gastritis (12.67%), itching without rash (1.3%), itching with rash (1.3%), arthralgia (2.67%), peripheral neuropathy (1.3%), drowsiness (1.3%), hepatotoxicity (2%), ototoxicity (0.67%)
Verma (2014)	India	118	May 2013–May 2014	DOTS	6	4	38.14	Raised liver transaminases (33.33%), nausea and vomiting (28.88%), hepatitis (20%), headache (20%), rash (20%), constipation (13.33%), fever (13.33%), flu-like syndrome (13.33%), blurred vision and optic neuritis (11.11%), hyperglycemia (11.11%), diarrhea (8.88%), peripheral neuritis (4.44%), arthralgia with increased blood uric acid level (4.44%), pruritis (4.44%), peripheral neuritis (4.44%), increased blood urea (2.22%), and urinary complaints like dysuria (2.22%)

Contd...

Contd...

Study year	Location	Sample size	Study period	Type of regimen	Duration of treatment (months)	Number of drugs in regimens	Incidence of ADRs (%)	Profile of ADRs
Farazi (2014)	Iran	940	May 2010–Mar 2014	DOTS	6–9	5	Major – 5.8 Minor – 22.8	Hepatobiliary system (35.7%), gastrointestinal tract (22%), musculoskeletal system (19.5%), skin and appendages (15.3%), peripheral nervous systems (3%), hematologic system (1.2%), ototoxicity (1.2%), visual system (1.1%), renal system (0.9%)
Sivaraj (2014)	India	100	Jun 2003–Feb 2006	DOTS and Non-DOTS (50 each)	6–12	5	Group 1–58 Group 2–132	Group 1 – GIT (16%), Hepatotoxicity (8%), Hematological toxicity (8%), Dermatitis (12%), fever/flu like symptoms/arthralgia/gout (14%) group 2 – git (32%), hepatotoxicity (24%) hematological toxicity (24%), dermatitis (16%), optic neuritis (4%), ototoxicity (2%), fever/flu like symptoms/arthralgia/gout (30%)
Athira (2015)	India	511	Jul 2013–Nov 2013	DOTS	6–9	5	18.20	Gastrointestinal problem (38.09%), skin reaction (30.48%), hepatotoxicity (14.28%), arthralgia with hyperuricemia (1.90%), hearing problem (0.95%), vision problem (0.95%)

Note: Many authors have quoted different terminologies for describing various adverse drug reactions associated with anti-tuberculosis drugs. Therefore, these terminologies have been retained as described in above mentioned studies published by the authors.

GASTROINTESTINAL ADRS

Gastrointestinal symptoms are one of the most common ADRs seen with intake of antitubercular drugs. Its severity can range from mild symptoms like nausea, vomiting to life-threatening complications. All the first-line antitubercular drugs can cause mild gastrointestinal upsets that can be managed symptomatically without change in dosage of drugs. In a study of 893 patients by Shinde et al., it was found that gastrointestinal upset with nausea, vomiting, and abdominal pain were the most common ADRs seen in 12.5% of patients. In another prospective study from China, it was found that gastrointestinal ADRs were seen in 3.74% of 4304 patients and only 7 patients required hospital admissions.

HEPATOTOXICITY

The clinical presentation of ATT-associated hepatitis is similar to that of acute viral hepatitis. ATT-induced hepatotoxicity can manifest as transitory asymptomatic rise in transaminases or acute liver failure. The frequency of hepatotoxicity ranges from 2% to 39% in different countries. An increased incidence of hepatotoxicity has been observed in Indian sub-population when compared to Western population. ATT-induced hepatotoxicity in Indian population was observed to be 11.5%. However, a meta-analysis in West found the risk to be 4–28%. The occurrence of drug-induced hepatotoxicity is unpredictable though certain patients are at a relatively higher risk than other populations. The incidence has been reported to be higher in developing countries and factors such as acute or chronic liver disease, indiscriminate use of drugs, malnutrition and more advanced TB have been implicated. Isolated isoniazid administration resulted in a threefold increase in alanine aminotransferase levels over the normal in 10–20% of these patients. A meta-analysis of six studies investigating the use of isoniazid in isolation reported the incidence of hepatitis to be 0.6%. However, recent studies have observed the incidence of clinical hepatitis in patients receiving isoniazid to be lower than previously thought. Hepatotoxicity is rare in children receiving Isoniazid (INH). In a 10-year retrospective analysis, the incidence of hepatotoxicity in 564 children receiving INH for the prophylactic treatment of tuberculosis was observed as 0.18%. The incidence of hepatotoxicity was observed to be more in children receiving both INH and rifampicin. In a retrospective study of 430 children treated with both INH and rifampicin, hepatotoxicity was observed in 3.3%. Transitory and asymptomatic increases in the serum levels of bilirubin and hepatic enzymes occurred in 5% of patients with rifampicin. When isoniazid was used in combination with rifampicin, the incidence of hepatitis was observed to be 2.7%. Cholestatic hepatitis occurred in 2.7% of the patients receiving rifampicin in combination with Isoniazid and was 1.1% when rifampicin was received in combination with ATT other than

Isoniazid. Pyrazinamide is the most hepatotoxic of the drugs. Studies from Nepal reported the incidence of hepatotoxicity in patients receiving ATT to range from as 8% to 35%. In a study in Pakistan, it was found that ATT-induced hepatotoxicity was seen in 67 (19.76%) out of 339 patients and was seen more common in smear AFB-negative patients. However, incidence of hepatotoxicity from studies from Brazil and Japan was similar to Indian population. The risk of hepatotoxicity from ATT drugs was influenced by clinical and genetic factors. In a study done by Singh et al., ATT-induced hepatotoxicity presented as jaundice in 61% patients followed by prodromal symptoms in 39% and life-threatening complications in 16.6%. Studies have also observed that 0.01% of patients taking ATT are at a risk of developing Acute liver failure (ALF) and the contribution of ATT in magnitude of ALF population may be even higher in countries in which tuberculosis as well as hepatitis virus(es) are endemic. In the study conducted in nearly 1200 acute liver patients in India, ATT was the cause in 5.6% of cases and three-fourths (76%) of ATT-ALF patients died within 5 days of hospitalization.

PERIPHERAL NEUROPATHY

Peripheral neuropathy occurs in approximately 20% of patients treated with isoniazid. This was similar to findings of a study in Pakistan where peripheral neuropathy characterized by tingling and burning sensation in the hands and feet was the most common ADR observed with isoniazid. The other anti-TB drug known to cause peripheral neuropathy is ethambutol, but very rare in comparison to isoniazid. In a study conducted by Koju et al., peripheral neuropathy was experienced by only 18.57% of the patients. In the existing literatures also, occurrence of peripheral neuropathy is considered rare with the recommended doses of isoniazid used in DOTS strategy. In a study of 893 patients by Shinde et al., on patients started on first-line ATT, it was observed that 5.04% of patients had peripheral neuropathy and 0.22% had acute psychosis.

PSYCHIATRIC DISORDERS

Isoniazid-related psychiatric disorders can manifest as psychosis, obsessive-compulsive neurosis, and mania, loss of memory and death. The first description of psychotic symptoms due to isoniazid was by Mandel et al., who reported three such cases in 1956. The mechanism of production of isoniazid-related psychiatric disorders is not clearly known, but isoniazid is known to interfere with several metabolic processes essential for the normal functioning of the neuron. Isoniazid causes deficiency of vitamin B6 by causing excessive excretion of the vitamin, which in turn leads to a disturbance of normal tryptophan metabolism. There is great variability in the clinical features of isoniazid-induced psychosis in the various reported cases. Jackson, in 1957, reported five cases of isoniazid-induced psychosis that presented with excessive argumentation, mental depression, euphoria, grandiose ideas, and complex delusions; none of these patients had any previous history of mental illness. Agarwala et al. reported symptoms of restlessness, irritability, emotional instability, agitation, apprehension, and fluctuation in behavior after isoniazid therapy. Bedi et al. reported a case of isoniazid psychosis in a 74-year-old, who developed restlessness, irritability, aimless activity, and incongruous actions 10 days after starting isoniazid therapy. Tiwari et al. reported a case of Isoniazid-induced psychosis with disturbed sleep, restlessness, and abnormal behavior. The durations of psychotic symptoms in these case reports varied widely, i.e. 7–45 days, 7 days, 10 days, and 120 days. A review of all cases of drug-induced seizures reported to the California Poison Control System revealed that of 386 cases, 23 (5.9%) were due to Isoniazid. In a study of 83 healthcare workers who received a 6-month course of Isoniazid, 34 (41%) developed an ADR. In 26 of these 34 patients, toxicity resulted in discontinuance of therapy. Toxic psychosis developed while under treatment with Isoniazid in 5 cases seen at Louisiana. In Peru, severe psychiatric syndrome occurred in approximately 1% of tuberculosis cases between 1991 and 1999. In Turkey, out of 1149 patients with established tuberculosis who initially received ATT therapy, neuropsychiatric manifestations were observed in 0.7% of patients.

RETROBULBAR NEURITIS

Ethambutol is one of the important first-line drugs in the treatment of tuberculosis. Carr and Henkind et al. first described the ocular ADRs of Ethambutol therapy in 1962. Retro-bulbar neuritis is the most important potential ADR from Ethambutol. It is reversible in most cases and is related to the dose and duration of treatment, but may occasionally become irreversible resulting in permanent visual disability, especially in the older population. The reported incidence of retro-bulbar neuritis when ethambutol is taken for more than 2 months is 18% in subjects receiving greater than 35 mg/kg/day, 5–6% with 25 mg/kg/day, and less than 1% with 15 mg/kg/day.

OTOTOXICITY

Streptomycin predominantly affects the vestibular system. Audiometry data suggest that the incidence of ototoxicity may be as high as 25%. Prazic and Salaj et al. found audiologically defined lesions in 36% of a group of 975 children treated with streptomycin sulfate for pulmonary tuberculosis. Hearing loss has also been reported in infants of tuberculous mothers treated with streptomycin during pregnancy. Familial occurrence of drug-induced toxicity has also been reported. In a large Indian study with short course chemotherapy regimes in the treatment of patients with pulmonary tuberculosis, 16.1% of the patients given streptomycin developed vertigo which was severe in 5% cases. In 10% of these patients, the drug had to be stopped. Reduction of dosage was needed in about 20%. In another series of 1744 patients treated with various ATT, 10.3% developed intolerance to streptomycin. Involvement of the VIII cranial nerve was the most common (46.8%) untoward reaction. Neff et al. reported intolerance to streptomycin in 12.9% of their cases. In this series, also, vestibular and auditory dysfunction was the most common.

IMMUNOLOGICAL AND HEMATOLOGICAL ADRS

In a Brazilian study, Rifampicin-induced thrombocytopenia, leukopenia, eosinophilia, hemolytic anemia, agranulocytosis, vasculitis, acute interstitial nephritis, and septic shock occurred in 0.1% of the patients. However, few Asian studies reported allergic reactions with first-line ATT to be between 2.02% and 2.35% and hematological adverse effects to be 0.1–0.7%. Author in his work on hematological abnormalities during ATT found that thrombocytopenia, characterized by a rapid lowering of the platelet count in sensitive individuals was observed. Generally, the most common offending agent for the causation of thrombocytopenia secondary to antitubercular drugs is rifampicin. Isolated case reports showing thrombocytopenia following administration of pyrazinamide, isoniazid, ethambutol are found in literature and are attributed to an immunological phenomenon. Streptomycin is very rarely implicated as a cause of thrombocytopenia. Kant et al. reported thrombocytopenia secondary to rifampicin, ethambutol, and pyrazinamide in a single individual.

ARTHRALGIA

Pyrazinamide and ethambutol are two anti-tuberculous drugs that have been reported to induce hyperuricemia in non-gouty patients leading to arthralgia. The metabolite pyrazinoic acid is likely responsible for the hyperuricemic effect. The mechanism is related to pyrazinoic acid, the principal metabolite of pyrazinamide oxidized by xanthine oxidase, which inhibits the renal tubular secretion of uric acid. Hyperuricemia has been reported in 43–100% of patients treated with pyrazinamide (alone or in combination). Gouty attacks have also been associated with patients taking pyrazinamide. Ethambutol can also cause hyperuricemia by decreasing renal uric acid clearance, but it does so less consistently and to a lesser degree than pyrazinamide. In a study by Dhingra et al. on patients receiving DOTS therapy general aches and pains were complained by about 35%. However, in a study by Shinde et al., arthralgia was seen in0.67% which was lower incomparison to reported incidence of 2.57% in Chinese patients receiving ATT.

RENAL TOXICITY

Aminoglycosides produce renal toxic effects due to their accumulation in the renal tubules. Such effects are more common in elderly individuals and in patients with a history of kidney disease. The risk of nephrotoxicity is less and range around 2% while using streptomycin.

CUTANEOUS ADRS (CADRS)

Pyrazinamide has been described to cause various skin reactions like maculopapular rash, erythema multiforme, exfoliative dermatitis, and DRESS syndrome. Among the first-line drugs, pyrazinamide is the commonest cause of CADR (2.38%), followed by streptomycin (1.45%), ethambutol (1.44%), rifampicin (1.23%), and isoniazid (0.98%). It is not uncommon for exfoliative dermatitis to occur with more than one of the four drugs. It is unclear whether renal failure predisposes to increased occurrence of CADRs. So far, no definite association exists between pre-existing renal insufficiency and increased incidence of CADRs. The incidence of ethambutol induced rash is found to be 0.5%. The author reported a rare occurrence of exfoliative dermatitis secondary to ethambutol and pyrazinamide in a 18-year-old female. Patients receiving Isoniazid can develop antinuclear antibodies during the use of the drug. Less than 1% develops systemic lupus erythematosus, the incidence of which is the same in both genders. Isoniazid administration can also worsen pre-existing lupus.

OTHER ADRS

Few case reports on Isoniazid-induced gynecomastia among patients treated with ATT. A rare occurrence of anaphylactic shock due to streptomycin was also reported.

CONCLUSION

The treatment of tuberculosis can cause a variety of ADRs. Accurate diagnoses and knowledge of the pharmacological properties of the drugs involved will allow professionals to tailor their approach to each individual case in near future.

FURTHER READINGS

1. Agarwala MC, Kansal HM, Gupta RK, Gupta DK, Kumar S. Toxic psychosis due to isoniazid. Indian J Tuberc. 1975;3:119-20.
2. Anand AC, Seth AK, Paul M, Puri P. Risk factors of hepatotoxicity during anti-tuberculosis treatment. MJAFI. 2006;62:45-9.

3. Athira B, Manju CS, Jyothi E. A study on adverse drug reactions to first line anti-tubercular drugs in DOTS therapy. Int J Pharmacol Clin Sci. 2015;4:7-11.
4. Baghaei P, Tabarsi P, Chitsaz E, et al. Incidence, clinical and epidemiological risk factors, and outcome of drug-induced hepatitis due to antituberculous agents in new tuberculosis cases. Am J Ther. 2010;17:17-22.
5. Carr RE, Henkind P. Ocular manifestations of ethambutol. Arch Ophthalmol. 1962;67:566-71.
6. Chhetri AK, Saha A, Verma SC, Palaian S, Mishra P, Shankar PR. A study of adverse drug reactions caused by first line anti-tubercular drugs used in Directly Observed Treatment, Short course (DOTS) therapy in western Nepal, Pokharan. J Pak Med Assoc. 2008;58:531-6.
7. Citron KM, Thomas GO. Ocular toxicity from ethambutol (editorial). Thorax. 1986;41:737-9.
8. Dalal NP, Karandikar YS, Pandit VA. Safety evaluation of directly observed treatment short course (DOTS) regimen in a tertiary care hospital, Pune. Int J Basic Clin Pharmacol. 2014;3:369-76.
9. de Jager P, van Altena R. Hearing loss and nephrotoxicity in long-term aminoglycoside treatment in patients with tuberculosis. Int J Tuberc Lung Dis. 2002;6:622-27.
10. Dhingra VK, Rajpal S, Aggarwal N, Aggarwal JK, Shadab K, Jain SK. Adverse drug reactions observed during DOTS. J Commun Dis. 2004;36:251-9.
11. Dosumu A. Side effects of drugs used in directly observed treatment short-course in newly diagnosed pulmonary tuberculosis subjects in Nigerian's: a controlled clinical study. Niger Post Grad Med J. 2002;9:34-7.
12. Durand F, Bernuau J, Pessayre D, et al. Deleterious influence of pyrazinamide on the outcome of patients with fulminant or subfulminant liver failure during antituberculous treatment including isoniazid. Hepatology. 1995;21:929-32.
13. Edwards R, Aronson JK. Adverse drug reactions: definitions, diagnosis, and management. Lancet. 2000;356:1255-9.
14. Forget EJ, Menzies D. Adverse reactions to first-line anti-tuberculosis drugs. Expert Opin Drug Saf. 2006;5:231-49.
15. Gangadharan PRJ. Isoniazid, rifampicin and hepatotoxicity. Am J Respir Dis. 1986;133:963-65.
16. Garg R, Gupta V, Mehra S, Singh R, Prasad R. Rifampicin induced thrombocytopenia. Indian J Tuberc. 2007;54:94-6.
17. Garg R, Mehra S, Prasad R. Isoniazid induced gynaecomastia: a case report. Indian J Tuberc. 2009;56:51-54.
18. Garg R, Verma S, Mahajan V, Prasad R. Exfoliative dermatitis secondary to ethambutol and pyrazinamide. Internet J Pulm Med. 2008;9:1.
19. Gholami K, Kamali E, Hajiabdolbagh M, Shalviri G. Evaluation of anti-tuberculosis induced adverse reactions in hospitalized patients. Pharm Pract. 2006;4:134-8.
20. Gutman AB, Yu TF, Berger L. Renal function in gout. III. Estimation of tubular secretion and reabsorption of uric acid by use of pyrazinamide (pyrazinoic acid). Am J Med. 1969;47:575-92.
21. Gülbay BE, Gürkan Ö, Yildiz Ö, et al. Side effects due to primary anti-tuberculosis drugs during the initial phase of therapy in 1149 hospitalized patients for tuberculosis. J Respir Med. 2006;10:1834-42.
22. Jain VK, Vardhar H, Prakash OM. Pyrazinamide induced thrombocytopenia. Tubercle. 1988;69:217-8.
23. Jeong JI, Jung BH, Kim MH, Lim JM, Ha DC, Cho SW. The influence of adverse drug reactions on first-line anti-tuberculosis chemotherapy in the elderly patients. Tuberc Respir Dis. 2009;67:325-30.

24. Kant S, Verma K, Gupta V, Anand SC, Prasad R. Pyrazinamide induced thrombocytopenia. Indian J Pharmacol. 2010;42:108-9.
25. Khadka J, Malla P, Jha SS, Poudel SR. The study of drug induced hepatotoxicity in ATT patients attending in National Tuberculosis Center in Bhaktapur, SAARC. J Tuber Lung Dis HIV/AIDS. 2009;2:17-21.
26. Kishore PV, Palaian S, Ojha P, Shankar PR. Pattern of adverse drug reactions experienced by tuberculosis patients in a tertiary care teaching hospital in Western Nepal Pak. J Pharm Sci. 2008;21:51-6.
27. Koju D, Rao BS, Shrestha B, Shakya R, Makaju R. Occurrence of side effects from anti-tuberculosis drugs in urban Nepalese population under DOTS treatment. Kathmandu Univ J Sci Eng Technol. 2005;1.
28. Kumar R, Shalimar. Bhatia V, et al. Anti-tuberculosis therapy-induced acute liver failure: magnitude, profile, prognosis, and predictors of outcome. Hepatology. 2010;51:1665-74.
29. Kurniawati F, Sulaiman SAS, Gillani SW. Adverse drug reactions of primary anti-tuberculosis drugs among tuberculosis patients treated in chest clinic. Int J Pharm Life Sci. 2012;3:1331-8.
30. Lee AM, Mennone JZ, Jones RC, Paul WS. Risk factors for hepatotoxicity associated with rifampin and pyrazinamide for the treatment of latent tuberculosis infection: experience from three public health tuberculosis clinics. Int J Tuberc Lung Dis. 2002;6:995-1000.
31. Lv X, Tang S, Xia Y, et al. Adverse reactions due to directly observed treatment strategy therapy in Chinese tuberculosis patients: a prospective study. PLOS ONE. 2013;8:e65037. http://dx.doi.org/10.1371/journal.pone.0065037.
32. Maciel ELN, Guidoni LM, Favero JL, et al. Adverse effects of the new tuberculosis treatment regimen recommended by the Brazilian National Ministry of Health. J Bras Pneumol. 2010;36:232-8.
33. Mandal PK, Mandal A, Bhattacharyya SK. Comparing the daily versus the intermittent regimens of the anti-tubercular chemotherapy in the initial intensive phase in non-HIV, sputum positive, pulmonary tuberculosis patients. J Clin Diagn Res. 2013;7:292-5.
34. Moore RE, Smith CR, Lietman PS:. Risk factors for the development of auditory toxicity in patients receiving aminoglycosides. J Infect Dis. 1984;149:23-30.
35. Neff TA, Coan BJ. Incidence of drug intolerance to antituberculosis chemotherapy. Dis Chest. 1969;56:10-2.
36. Pande JN, Singh SPN, Khilnani GC, Tandon RK. Risk factors for hepatotoxicity from antituberculous drugs: a case control study. Thorax. 1996;51:132-6.
37. Parthasarathy R, Sarma GR, Janardhanam B, et al. Hepatic toxicity in south Indian patients during treatment of tuberculosis with short-course regimens containing isoniazid, rifampicin and pyrazinamide. Tubercle. 1986;67:99-108.
38. Postlethwaite AE, Bartel AG, Kelley WN. Hyperuricemia due to ethambutol. N Engl J Med. 1972;286:761-62.
39. Prasad R, Garg R, Verma SK. Isoniazid- and ethambutol-induced psychosis. Ann Thorac Med. 2008;3:149-51.
40. Prasad R, Mukerji PK. Rifampicin induced thrombocytopenia. Indian J Tuberc. 1989;36:171-5.
41. Prasad R, Mukherji PK. Ethambutol induced thrombocytopenia. Tubercle. 1989;70:211-2.
42. Prasad R. Anaphylactic shock due to streptomycin sulphate. J Indian Med Assoc. 1989;82:254-5.
43. Rakotoson JL, Randriamanana D, Rakotomizao JR, Andrianasolo R, Rakotoarivelo R, Andrianarisoa AC. Severe systemic lupus erythematosus induced by isoniazid [Article in French]. Rev Pneumol Clin. 2009;65:361-64.

44. Rybak MJ, Abate BJ, Kang SL, Ruffing MJ, Lerner SA, Drusano GL. Prospective evaluation of the effect of an aminoglycoside dosing regimen on rates of observed nephrotoxicity and ototoxicity. Antimicrob Agents Chemother. 1999;43:1549-55.
45. Shakya R, Rao BS. Incidence of hepatotoxicity due to antitubercular medicines and assessment of risk factors. Ann Pharmacother. 2004;38:1074-9.
46. Sharma SK, Balamurugan A, Saha PK, Pandey RM, Mehra NK. Evaluation of clinical and immunogenetic risk factors for the development of hepatotoxicity during antituberculosis treatment. Am J Respir Crit Care Med. 2002;166:916-9.
47. Shinde KM, Pore SM, Bapat TR. Adverse reactions to first-line anti-tuberculous agents in hospitalised patients: pattern, causality, severity and risk factors. Indian J Med Spec. 2013;4:1-4.
48. Singla R, Sharma SK, Mohan A, et al. Evaluation of risk factors for antituberculosis treatment-induced hepatotoxicity. Indian J Med Res. 2010;132:81-6.
49. Sinha K, Marak IR, Singh WA. Adverse drug reactions in tuberculosis patients due to directly observed treatment strategy therapy: experience at an outpatient clinic of a teaching hospital in the city of Imphal, Manipur. Indian J Assoc Chest Phys. 2013;1:50-3.
50. Steele MA, Burk RF, Desprez RM. Hepatitis with isoniazid and rifampicin – a meta analysis. Chest. 1971;99:465-71.
51. Tan WC, Ong CK, Lo Kang SC, Abdul Razak M. Two years review of cutaneous adverse drug reaction from first line anti-tuberculous drugs. Med J Malaysia. 2007;62:143-6.
52. Tsai RK, Lee YH. Reversibility of ethambutol optic neuropathy. J Ocul Pharmacol Ther. 1997;13:473-7.
53. Verma R, Mahor GR, Shrivastava AK, Pathak P. Adverse drug reactions associated with first line anti-tubercular drugs in a tertiary care hospital of central India: a study of clinical presentations, causality, and severity. Asian J Pharm Clin Res. 2014;7:140-3.
54. Vieira DE, Gomes M. Adverse effects of tuberculosis treatment: experience at an outpatient clinic of a teaching hospital in the city of São Paulo, Brazil. J Bras Pneumol. 2008;34:1049-55.
55. World Health Organization. Requirements for Adverse Reaction Reporting. Geneva, Switzerland: World Health Organization; 1975.
56. Yee D, Valiquette C, Pelletier M, Parisien I, Rocher I, Menzies D. Incidence of serious side effects from first-line anti-tuberculosis drugs among patients treated for active tuberculosis. Am J Respir Crit Care Med. 2003;167:1472-7.

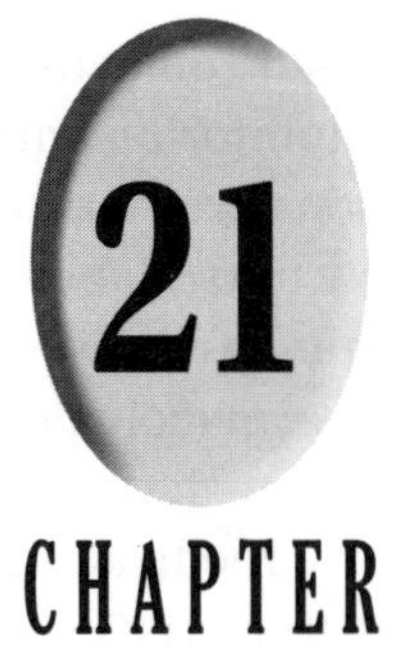

CHAPTER

Epidemiology of Adverse Drug Reactions with Second Line Drugs among Patients Treated for Multidrug Resistant Tuberculosis

Multidrug resistant TB (MDR-TB) is defined as *M. tuberculosis* resistant to isoniazid and rifampicin with or without resistance to other first line drugs. It is considered to be a worldwide problem with notoriously difficult and challenging treatment. The emergence of resistance to drugs used to treat tuberculosis, and particularly MDR-TB, has become a significant public health problem in a number of countries and an obstacle to effective tuberculosis control. The prevalence of MDR-TB among notified new and re-treatment pulmonary tuberculosis patients are estimated to be 3.5% and 20.5% respectively. Patients may present with a variety of adverse drug reactions when second line drugs (SLDs) are prescribed for MDR-TB management. Most of adverse drug reactions are minor and can be managed without discontinuation of treatment. Some adverse drug reactions can be life-threatening if not recognized and treated promptly. There are major concerns regarding SLDs in that they are expensive, have low efficacy and more toxic as compared to first line antituberculosis drugs. Adverse drug reactions associated with SLDs can have severe impact on efficient management. There may be a severe impact on adherence and higher risk of default and treatment failure affecting outcome overall if such adverse drug reactions are not properly managed. This review aims to highlight the prevalence of adverse drug reactions in patients receiving SLDs for treatment of MDR-TB.

PREVALENCE OF ADVERSE DRUG REACTIONS AMONG PATIENTS RECEIVING SLDS: GLOBAL

The management of MDR-TB patients has been considered to be complicated and challenging because of prolonged duration of 24 to 27 months of treatment and high toxicity profile of SLDs. The prevalence of adverse drug reactions observed in various studies conducted worldwide ranged from 69%–96%. The reasons for the difference in the prevalence of adverse drug reactions across these studies might be related to several possible factors such as: differences in definitions of adverse drug reactions terminologies as adopted by physicians, whether the adverse drug reactions were reported by patient (subjective) or detected by clinician (objective) on the basis of clinical evidence along with feasibility of monitoring with serial laboratory investigations, whether all or only the major adverse drug reactions were studied, the differences in comorbidities such as diabetes and other covariates including HIV coinfection and variations in the use of specific antitubercular drugs including dosage and also pharmacological interactions with other group of drugs comprising antiretroviral, oral hypoglycemic agents in case of diabetics and also ancillary medications used for management of adverse drug reactions. The characteristics of various studies showing frequency of adverse drug reactions are shown in Table 21.1. The observed frequency of specific gastrointestinal adverse drug reactions has been reported in 0.5–100% patients. The high prevalence of gastrointestinal adverse drug reactions in few of the studies was probably due to frequent reporting by patients as compared to other adverse drug reactions leading to subjective variation. Ototoxicity has been reported in 12–70% patients receiving SLDs. The frequency of tinnitus has been reported in 5–45% patients, while that of deafness is reported in 6.7–33% patients. Ototoxicity is predominantly associated with the use of injectable aminoglycoside (Kanamycin) although there is possibility of additive effects of interaction with other concomitant and potentially ototoxic drugs that were used in the regimen such as ofloxacin and cycloserine. This warrants further investigation to uncover the possibility of these interactive effects. Several studies have highlighted regarding high potential of these SLDs to cause adverse drug reactions that has led to interruption of treatment in 19–60% of MDR-TB patients. This high prevalence may be due to early identification and aggressive management strategies adopted by DOTS PLUS program. Baghaei et al. reported deafness and headache/psychosis occurring due to injectable kanamycin and cycloserine respectively as major adverse drug reactions that required frequent discontinuation and/or substitution. MDR-TB patients should be managed aggressively for adverse drug reactions during therapy, especially for ototoxicity and psychiatric disorders.

PREVALENCE OF ADVERSE DRUG REACTIONS AMONG PATIENTS RECEIVING SLDS: INDIA

Very few have especifically reported frequency of adverse drug reactions in India. A study conducted in Tamil Nadu by Joseph P et. al. reported adverse drug reactions in 86.8% patients. Only 5 patients did not complain of any adverse drug reactions. Adverse drug reactions were considered mild if the patient made 1 or 2 complaints during the 12 month period and only required symptomatic treatment, moderate if the complaint was repeated or of prolonged duration but still could be managed with symptomatic drugs,

TABLE 21.1: Characteristics of important studies showing frequency of adverse drug reactions due to second line drugs

Study Year	Location	Sample size	Study period	HIV prevalance (%)	Age (years)	History of previous treatment	Type of regimen used	Length of treatment (months)	Number of drugs used	Number of patients experiencing atleast one adverse drug reaction	Adverse drug reactions most frequently observed	Incidence of major adverse drug reactions (%)	Mortality observed due to major adverse drug reactions
Tahaoglu (2001)	Turkey	158	1992–1999	NA	15–68	80	Individualized	26.5 (24–30)	14	64	Ototoxicity	39	Nil
Furin (2001)	Peru	60	1996–1998	1.7	26	100	Individualized	20 (6–25)	8	60	Gastrointestinal	11.7	Nil
Nathanson (2004)	Estonia, Latvia, Peru, Phillippines, Russia	818	1998–2002	NA	NA	NA	Individualized	34 (24–42)	10	NA	Gastrointestinal	32.1	Nil
Prasad (2006)	India	46	1998–2002	NA	30.2	100	Standardized	24 (17–32)	6	16	Gastrointestinal	21.1	Nil
Shin (2007)	Russia	244	2000–2002	NA	32.5	100	Individualized	18.5 (1–42.4)	14	73.3	Gastrointestinal	28.7	Nil
Masjedi (2008)	Iran	43	2002–2006	NA	44.4	100	Standardized	24	8	25	Ototoxicity	46.5	Yes
Seung (2009)	South Africa	76	2007–2008	74	35	97	Standardized and individualized	24	6	70	Neurological	NA	Nil
Singla (2009)	India	126	2002–2006	NA	26	100	Standardized	24	6	73	Gastrointestinal	18	Nil
Bloss (2010)	Latvia	1027	2000–2004	3.1	41.2	63	Individualized	18–24	6	807	Gastrointestinal	84	Nil

Contd...

Contd...

Study Year	Location	Sample size	Study period	HIV prevalance (%)	Age (years)	History of previous treatment	Type of regimen used	Length of treatment (months)	Number of drugs used	Number of patients experiencing atleast one adverse drug reaction	Adverse drug reactions most frequently observed	Incidence of major adverse drug reactions (%)	Mortality observed due to major adverse drug reactions
Van Deun (2010)	Bangladesh	427	1997–2007	NA	33.8	87.1	Standardized	15 (9–21)	8	47.5	Gastrointestinal	4.2	Nil
Baghaei (2011)	Iran	80	2006–2009	5	40.6	100	Standardized	24	6	45	Ototoxicity	15	Yes
Joseph (2011)	India	38	2006–2007	NA	30-45	100	Standardized	24	6	33	Gastrointestinal	58	Nil
Sagwa (2012)	Namibia	59	2008–2010	53	34.7	92	Individualized	24	15	90	Gastrointestinal	73	Nil
Caroll (2012)	Korea	655	2005–2009	NA	NA	51.5	Individualized	28 (25–31)	19	NA	Gastrointestinal	16	Nil
Isaakidis (2012)	India	67	2007–2011	100	35.5	92.5	Individualized and standardized	10 (1–30)	15	71 (Mild) 63 (Mod.)	Gastrointestinal	59.7	Nil
Jacobs (2012)	South Africa	350	2010–2011	72.6	35.7	NA	Standardized	24	6	282	Ototoxicity	NA	Nil
Van der Walt (2013)	South Africa	2079	2000–2004	66.8	36.3	90.6	Standardized	19 (16–22)	8	66.8	Ototoxicity	6	Nil
Bezu (2014)	Ethiopia	73	2012–2013	No	28	87.7	Individualized	24	6	73	Gastrointestinal	NA	Nil

and severe if either a reduction of dosage or termination of the offending drug(s) was warranted. Severe adverse drug reactions were observed in 58% patients. Of these, 13 had termination of ethionamide, 4 of ofloxacin, and 1 each had kanamycin, ethambutol, pyrazinamide or cycloserine terminated. In addition, ofloxacin dosage was reduced in 1 patient, pyrazinamide in 2 others, and kanamycin injections changed to 3 days a week in 5 patients.

Another study conducted in Mumbai among 67 HIV/MDR-TB coinfected patients were being treated with anti-TB treatment and anti-retroviral therapy reported that overall adverse drug reactions were common. In this cohort, 71%, 63% and 40% of patients experienced one or more mild, moderate or severe adverse drug reactions respectively. However, they were rarely life-threatening or debilitating. Adverse drug reactions occurring most frequently included gastrointestinal symptoms (45%), peripheral neuropathy (38%), hypothyroidism (32%), psychiatric symptoms (29%) and hypokalemia (23%). Eleven patients were hospitalized for adverse drug reactions and one or more suspect drugs had to be permanently discontinued in 40% patients. No adverse drug reactions led to indefinite suspension of an entire MDR-TB or ART regimen. One study conducted at Delhi reported that 40% patients experienced minor adverse drug reactions, defined as those requiring either no discontinuation of a drug or discontinuation for <1 week and manageable at peripheral level. 22 (18%) patients had major adverse drug reactions requiring treatment modification. PAS was used in 46 patients: 6 patients (5%) developed simple goiter, which responded to thyroxin replacement therapy with continuation of PAS. In 15 (12%) patients, cycloserine had to be stopped due to major psychotic reactions varying from major depression, psychosis to violent behavior. Kanamycin was stopped in 5 (4%) patients due to hearing loss/ giddiness. Ofloxacin and pyrazinamide were stopped in one patient due to severe arthralgia, and pyrazinamide was stopped in another patient due to hepatotoxicity. All of these major adverse drug reactions required referral to specialist hospitals. None of the patients required discontinuation of the entire treatment regimen, although two patients defaulted due to adverse drug reactions. No deaths due to drug toxicity were recorded in the cohort. A study conducted at Lucknow by Prasad et. al. among MDR-TB patients treated with second line drugs and reported that overall 16 (41%) patients experienced adverse drug reactions. Seven patients complained of nausea and vomiting of which in three patients PAS was stopped after six to eight months of treatment, as it was thought to be the cause. The remaining patients did not require any change of medication. Four patients developed photosensitivity and sparfloxacin was replaced in one of the patients by ofloxacin after three months of treatment. In rest of the patients, it did not require any change of medication. Tinnitus and vertigo developed in four patients after one to five months of treatment due to kanamycin and it had to be stopped in two of them. Three patients developed depression and abnormal behavior possibly due to cycloserine, which was replaced by a quinolone in two patients. However, it was continued with anti-psychosis treatment in the remaining patient. A total of 21.1% patients suffered from significant adverse drug reactions, which required stoppage/change of drugs. No other adverse drug reactions, such as arthralgia or cardiotoxicity were observed in any patient. In other study, among 98 MDR-TB patients under modified DOTS PLUS treatment, it was observed that 43.9% patients experienced at least one adverse drug reactions. Adverse drug reaction observed most frequently were nausea/vomiting 24 (24.5%) patients, hearing disturbances 12 (12.3%) patients, dizziness/vertigo 10 (10.2%) patients and arthralgia 9 (9.2%) patients. 17 (17.4%) patients had major adverse drug reactions requiring change or stoppage of drugs that included ototoxicity (6.1%), headache and psychosis (4.1%), gastrointestinal intolerance and hypothyroidism (3.1%) as well as arthralgia and hepatitis (4.1%). Agents responsible for these adverse drug reactions were kanamycin (ototoxicity), cycloserine (headache/psychosis), ethionamide (gastrointestinal tolerance/hypothyroidism) and pyrazinamide (arthralgia/hepatitis). At the end of treatment 71 (72.4%) patients were treated successfully. There was no mortality due to occurrence of adverse drug reactions. Further studies are required for prevalence of adverse drug reaction in near future.

CONCLUSION

Adverse drug reactions of varying severity are common during treatment of MDR-TB, particularly in the intensive phase of therapy. Some adverse drug reactions were more prevalent in MDR-TB patients coinfected with HIV. Most adverse drug reactions can be successfully managed on an outpatient basis through a community-based treatment program, even in a resource-limited setting. Concerns about severe adverse drug reactions in the management of MDR-TB patients are justified, however, they should not cause delays in the urgently needed rapid scale-up of second-line anti-TB treatment. Adverse drug reactions can be detected by clinical evidence in resource-limited settings. MDR TB can be cured successfully with appropriate combination of drugs if adverse drug reactions associated with them can be managed aggressively and timely. Newer and less toxic drugs are urgently needed to treat MDR-TB patients.

FURTHER READINGS

1. Tahaoglu K, Torun T, Sevim T, Atac GB, Kir A, Karasulu L, et al. The treatment of MDR-TB in Turkey. N Engl J Med. 2001;345:170-4.
2. Furin JJ, Mitnick CD, Shin SS, Bayona J, Becerra MC, Singler JM, et al. Occurrence of serious adverse effects in patients receiving community-based therapy for MDR-TB. Int J tuberc Lung Dis. 2001;5:648-55.

3. Papastavros T, Dolovich LR, Holbrook A, Whitehead L, Loeb M. Adverse events associated with pyrazinamide and levofloxacin in the treatment of MDR-TB. CMAJ 2002;167:131-6.
4. Nathanson E, Gupta R., Huamani P, Leimane AD, Pasechnikov AD, Tupasi TE, et al. Adverse events in the treatment of MDR-TB: results from the DOTS-Plus initiative. Int J Tuberc Lung Dis. 2005;9:1027-33.
5. Törün T, Güngör G, Özmen I, Bölükba Y, Maden E, Bıçakçı B, et al. Side effects associated with the treatment of MDR-TB. Int J Tuberc Lung Dis. 2005;9:1373-7.
6. Nahar BL, Mosharrof Hossain AKM, Islam MM, Saha DR. A comparative study on the adverse effects of two anti-tuberculosis drugs regimen in initial two-month treatment period. Bangladesh J Pharmacol. 2006;1:51-7.
7. Shin SS, Pasechnikov AD, Gelmanova IY, Peremitin GG, Strelis AK, Mishustin S, et al. Adverse reactions among patients being treated for MDR-TB in Tomsk, Russia. Int J Tuberc Lung Dis. 2007;11:1314-20.
8. Lanternier F, Dalban C, Perez L, Bricaire F, Costagliola D, Caumes E. Tolerability of anti-tuberculosis treatment and HIV sero-status. Int J Tuberc Lung Dis. 2007;11:1203-9.
9. Bloss E, Kukša L, Holtz TH, Riekstina V, Skripconoka V, Kammerer S, et al. Adverse events related to MDR-TB treatment, Latvia, 2000-2004. Int J Tuberc Lung Dis. 2010;14:275-81.
10. Palmero D, Cruz V, Museli T, Pavlovsky H, Fernandez J, Waisman J. Adverse drug reactions in MDR-TB. Medicina (B Aires) 2010;70:427-33.
11. Baghaei P, Tabarsi P, Dorriz D, Marjani M, Shamaei M, Pooramiri MV, et al. Adverse effects of MDR-TB treatment with a standardized regimen: a report from Iran. Am J Ther. 2011;18:e29-34. doi: 10.1097/MJT.0b013e3181c0806d.
12. Carroll MW, Lee M, Cai Y, Hallahan CW, Shaw PA, Min JH, et al. Frequency of adverse reactions to first- and second-line anti-tuberculosis chemotherapy in a Korean cohort. Int J Tuberc Lung Dis 2012;167:961-66.http://dx.doi.org/10.5588/ijtld.11.0574
13. Sagwa E, Mantel-Teeuwisse AK, Ruswa N, Musasa JP, Pal S, Dhliwayo P, et al. The burden of adverse events during treatment of drug-resistant tuberculosis in Namibia. Southern Med Review. 2012;5:6-13.
14. Van der Walt M, Lancaster J, Odendaal R, Davis JG, Shean K. Serious Treatment Related Adverse Drug Reactions amongst Anti-Retroviral Naive MDR-TB Patients. PLoS ONE. 2013;8: e58817. doi:10.1371/journal.pone.0058817.
15. Singla R, Sarin R, Khalid UK, Mathuria K, Singla N. Seven-year DOTS-Plus pilot experience in India: results, constraints and issues. Int J Tuberc Lung Dis. 2009;13:976-81.
16. Joseph P, Desai VB, Mohan NS, Fredrick JS, Ramachandran R. Outcome of standardized treatment for patients with MDR-TB from Tamil Nadu, India. Indian J Med Res. 2011;133: 529-34.
17. Isaakidis P, Varghese B, Mansoor H, Cox HS, Ladomirska J. Adverse Events among HIV/MDR-TB Co-Infected Patients Receiving Antiretroviral and Second Line Anti-TB Treatment in Mumbai, India. PLoS ONE 2012;7:e40781. doi:10.1371/journal.pone.0040781.
18. Prasad R, Verma S K, S Sahai Kumar S Jain A. Efficacy and safety of kanamycin, ethionamide, PAS and cycloserine in multi drug resistant pulmonary tuberculosis patients. Indian J Chest Dis Allied Sci. 2006;48:181-4.
19. Prasad R, Singh A, Srivastav R, Hosmane GB, Kushwaha RAS, Jain A. Frequency of adverse events observed with second line drugs among patients treated for multidrug-resistant tuberculosis. Indian J Tub. 2016;63:106-14.

Index

A

P

Q

R

S

W

Z